KV-019-528

Questions and Answers on
Apley's *Concise System of Orthopaedics and Fractures*

C. B. D. LAVY, BSc, FRCS
Senior Registrar in Orthopaedics
Middlesex Hospital
London

D. S. BARRETT, BSc, FRCS
Clinical Lecturer in Orthopaedics
Institute of Orthopaedics
Royal National Orthopaedic Hospital
London

Foreword by A. Graham Apley

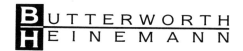

BUTTERWORTH
HEINEMANN

Butterworth-Heinemann Ltd
Linacre House, Jordan Hill, Oxford OX2 8DP

🌐 PART OF REED INTERNATIONAL BOOKS

OXFORD   LONDON   BOSTON
MUNICH   NEW DELHI   SINGAPORE   SYDNEY
TOKYO   TORONTO   WELLINGTON

First published 1991

© Butterworth-Heinemann Ltd 1991

British Library Cataloguing in Publication Data
Lavey, C.B.D.
Questions and answers on Apley's *Concise System
of Orthopaedics and Fractures.*
I. Title II. Barrett, D.S.
617.3   6200528493

ISBN 0 7506 1170 7

Library of Congress Cataloguing in Publication Data
A CIP record for this book is available from the British Library

Set by Cambridge Composing (UK) Ltd, Cambridge
Printed and bound in Great Britain by
Biddles Ltd, Guildford and King's Lynn

Contents

Foreword

When I was asked by the authors whether I would approve of a questions and answers book based on Apley's *Concise System of Orthopaedics and Fractures*, I was taken aback. Indeed, I consulted Professor Solomon, co-author of the book, before answering. I suppose that subconsciously I had assumed that the validity of our text was being questioned – and who likes to have the blemishes of his baby exposed? However, my conscious self (and Professor Solomon's reassurance) soon persuaded me that my Freudian fears were ill-founded. And, indeed, once I saw a few samples of the proposed work, I realized that it was based on the flattering assumption that our text was reliably accurate. Naturally, I no longer viewed the proposed work with a jaundiced eye, but I had to resist the temptation to apply my rose-tinted spectacles.

Nobody should doubt that the question and answer method is a very good way of learning and an excellent way of revising; it is the modern equivalent of the technique which Socrates used to such good effect. The questions in this book have been chosen with thoughtful discrimination and the answers are brief, lucid and informative. No undergraduate could fail to learn a great deal from them and a few postgraduates could fail to have their knowledge amplified and clarified; both are given the opportunity of numerical self-assessment which may sometimes be chastening but is always enlightening. Professor Solomon and I are proud to be associated with such a well-thought-out and helpful book.

A. Graham Apley

Preface

This short book of questions and answers was written to complement the popular *Concise System of Orthopaedics and Fractures* by Apley and Solomon, which we have used as the basis of our undergraduate teaching at the Middlesex Hospital and The Institute of Orthopaedics at the Royal National Orthopaedic Hospital, Stanmore. The questions are aimed primarily at medical students, physiotherapists and nurses specializing in orthopaedics. For this group of students, we have set an 'undergraduate target score' at the end of each chapter.

Postgraduate doctors studying for the second part of the new FRCS examination may also like to use the questions as a method of revision. For them, we would expect higher scores and we have also set a 'postgraduate target'.

The questions are arranged in chapters corresponding to the chapters in the *Concise System*; thus, a poor performance on any of the questions will usually be helped by reading the relevant section.

All growing specialities have controversial areas of great (and sometimes heated!) debate. Orthopaedics is no exception, and where there are a variety of ways of treating a condition, we have tended to stick to the method recommended in the *Concise System*.

C. B. D. Lavy
D. S. Barrett

Acknowledgements

Our thanks to Linda Skornia and Rosemary Dutton for typing the manuscript. We also thank Miss Gibson, Bob and Clare Woodwards and our undergraduate students for helpful suggestions.

How to use this book

The questions are on the left-hand page and the answers are opposite on the right. Use a card or a piece of paper to cover the answers while reading the questions.

The questions are of two types: either simple questions which require short answers, or statements which require a decision as to whether they are true or false. At the end of each question is a figure in brackets which represents the number of marks alloted to that question.

At the end of each chapter we have given target scores that might be expected of undergraduate and postgraduate readers.

Diagnosis in Orthopaedics

1. Pain in orthopaedic conditions is rarely referred. (1)

2. 'Diaphysis' refers to the shaft section of a long bone. (1)

3. Swelling of a joint occurring slowly is most likely to be due to an effusion rather than a haemarthrosis. (1)

4. Abduction is movement away from the body in the sagittal plane. (1)

5. Muscle imbalance causes weakness around joints, but not joint deformity. (1)

6. Varus deformity means the part of the limb distal to the joint is displaced towards the midline. (1)

7. Bone deformity may arise following growth plate injury (e.g. epiphyseal separation). (1)

8. Due to the splinting effect of the ribs, the thoracic spine is straight when viewed from the side. (1)

9. Radiographs which show osteophytes on the joint margins indicate rhematoid arthritis. (1)

10. Joint laxity occurs in 5% of people. (1)

11. Name four regions which classically exhibit hypermobility in lax jointed individuals. (2)

12. Multiple bony lumps are seen in von Recklinghausen's disease. (1)

Answers opposite

Diagnosis in Orthopaedics

1. False: pain arising from deep structures is often diffuse and poorly localized. This may be referred, for example the pain of sciatica which is referred to the thigh and leg.

2. True

3. True: haemarthrosis which is bleeding into a joint usually arises rapidly after injury.

4. False: abduction is movement away from the body in the *coronal* plane.

5. False: eventually, due to lack of balanced muscular support, joint deformity occurs.

6. True: valgus deformity is the opposite.

7. True: injury causing angulation or damage to part of the growth plate may result in deformity as the bone continues to elongate.

8. False: the thoracic spine has a kyphosis (convex posteriorly) of up to 40° in the normal adult. The ribs do, however, prevent excessive flexion/extension movements.

9. False: osteophyte formation is characteristic of osteoarthritis.

10. True: 5% of the population have hypermobile joints. This is often familial.

11. Any four from: fingers, thumb, spine, elbows, knees, wrist.

12. False: the lumps of von Recklinghausen's disease are neurofibromas and not bony. Bony lumps are seen in multiple exostoses (diaphyseal aclasis) and dyschondroplasia (Ollier's disease).

13. Give three radiological signs of osteoarthritis of a joint. (3)

14. Ankylosis is pathological fusion of a joint. (1)

15. Give two areas where CT scanning is of particular use in orthopaedics. (2)

16. Radionuclide scanning (scintigraphy) uses a radioactive bone-seeking iodine isotope. (1)

17. Increased uptake shown 3 hours after injection of isotope for bone scanning indicates new bone formation. (1)

18. Magnetic resonance imaging allows better differentiation of soft tissue than CT scanning. (1)

19. Computerized tomography (CT) allows effective cross-sectional imaging of metallic implants. (1)

20. Speed of nerve conduction in an average peripheral nerve is 40–60 metres per second. (1)

21. Velocity of conduction is increased by compression, which causes the nerve to become irritable. (1)

22. Galvanic stimulation of a muscle following division of the nerve to that muscle produces no response. (1)

Total score	26
Target score	
Postgraduate	23
Undergraduate	19

Answers opposite

13. Any three from: loss of joint space, cyst formation, osteo-phytes, joint line sclerosis.

14. True: ankylosis may be bony or fibrous in nature.

15. Any two from: spine (e.g. lumbar disc, herniation, spinal stenosis and spinal fractures), pelvic and acetabular fractures, complex intraarticular fractures, e.g. tibial plateau, bone tumours.

16. False: a technetium isotope (^{99m}Tc) is used for bone scanning. Iodine is not concentrated in the bone, but in the thyroid.

17. True: this is the 'bone phase'. Increased activity immediately (the blood phase) indicates bone hyperaemia.

18. True: better reconstruction of tissue images is therefore possible.

19. False: one drawback of CT scanning is the blurring artefact produced on films by metallic implants.

20. True: individual speeds vary depending on the size and myeli-nation of the nerve.

21. False: velocity is slowed. This can be shown by electrodiagnostic tests.

22. False: it does produce a response, but that response is abnormal.

Infection

1. Acute osteomyelitis is more common in adults than children. (1)

2. The commonest causal organism in acute osteomyelitis is beta haemolytic streptococcus. (1)

3. Patients with sickle cell disease are prone to develop shigella bone infections. (1)

4. In children the growth plate of a long bone often acts as a barrier to the spread of infection. (1)

5. The acute inflammatory reaction in a bone causes a decrease in intraosseous pressure. (1)

6. An involucrum is defined as a piece of devitalized bone acting as a foreign body. (1)

7. The clinical features of acute osteomyelitis are those of any acute infection, i.e. pain, swelling, warmth and loss of function. (1)

8. X-ray changes in acute osteomyelitis are usually apparent after 48 hours. (1)

9. Name two investigations that are helpful in suspected osteomyelitis. (2)

10. Early active and passive movement of the affected limb is essential in acute osteomyelitis. (1)

11. Name three precautions that are taken to avoid infection in orthopaedic surgery when implants are used. (3)

Answers opposite

6

Infection

1. False

2. False: it is *Staphylococcus aureus*.

3. False: they are prone to develop salmonella bone infections.

4. True: in infants this is not so, consequently the infection may spread to the joint.

5. False: there is an increase in pressure which causes severe pain and may obstruct blood flow.

6. False: this describes a sequestrum. An involucrum is a casing of new bone formed by the elevated periosteum. It may contain holes (cloacae). If a piece of involucrum becomes devitalized it may, like any piece of dead bone, act as a sequestrum.

7. True

8. False: there is usually no abnormality for 10 days, then there may be some mottled rarefaction of the metaphysis and elevation of the periosteum with new bone formation.

9. Any two from: raised erythrocyte sedimentation rate, leucocytosis, positive blood culture, increased activity on isotope bone scan. X-rays are usually unhelpful in early osteomyelitis.

10. False: exactly the opposite, rest is essential.

11. Clean environment, i.e. patient, surgeon and theatre (laminar air flow). Meticulous surgical technique. Prophylactic antibiotics.

12. Antibiotics are usually effective in chronic osteomyelitis. (1)

13. A Brodies abscess occurs in the diaphysis of a long bone. (1)

14. Name two sites where tuberculous osteomyelitis commonly occurs. (2)

15. The commonest cause of acute suppurative arthritis is *Staphylococcus aureus*. (1)

16. Cartilage is seldom damaged in suppurative arthritis. (1)

17. Synovial thickening and periarticular osteoporosis are rare findings in tuberculous arthritis. (1)

18. Treatment of tuberculous arthritis involves early surgical fusion of infected joints. (1)

Total score   22
Target score
    Postgraduate   20
    Undergraduate   17

Answers opposite

12. False: the nature of this condition is that bacteria are relatively protected in bone and fibrous tissue from the bloodstream and hence from blood-borne antibiotics. Treatment usually involves surgical clearance.

13. False: it occurs in the metaphysis.

14. The spine and the hip.

15. True: in children under 3, *Haemophilus influenzae* is also fairly common.

16. False: it is destroyed by bacterial and cellular enzymes. If this process is not arrested urgently, irreversible damage will occur.

17. False: they are both common.

18. False: the mainstay of treatment is chemotherapy. Arthrodesis should only be performed late when all disease activity has settled.

Rheumatic Disorders

1. Rheumatoid arthritis affects 3% of the population. (1)

2. Women are three times more commonly affected by rheumatoid arthritis than men. (1)

3. Rheumatoid arthritis is a systemic disease with a possible autoimmune basis. (1)

4. Arthritis of the rheumatoid type does not run in families. (1)

5. One of the autoantibodies produced by patients with rheumatoid arthritis is anti-IgG rheumatoid factor. This is essential for the definitive diagnosis of rheumatoid arthritis. (1) 75%

6. Rheumatoid arthritis primarily attacks the articular cartilage. (1)

7. Instability and deformity of joints occur at a late stage in rheumatoid arthritis. (1)

8. Rheumatoid nodules are characteristic lesions in rheumatoid arthritis consisting of the debris of destroyed articular cartilage. (1)

9. The lungs may also be affected in rheumatoid disease. (1)

   - pleurisy +
   - Pulmonary fibrosis

10. Rheumatoid nodules may occur in the eye. (1)

11. Early rheumatoid arthritis usually affects the large joints. (1)

12. The development of rheumatoid nodules is pathognomonic of rheumatoid arthritis. (1)

Answers opposite

Rheumatic Disorders

1. True

2. True

3. True: antigen antibody complexes are deposited in the joint, which after activation of complement gives rise to a local inflammatory reaction.

4. False: a genetically determined abnormal immune response may exist. Patients with rheumatoid arthritis show an increased frequency of the antigen HLA-DR4.

5. False: a negative test for IgG rheumatoid factor does not exclude rheumatoid arthritis.

6. False: the synovium is the primary site for the initial inflammatory changes of rheumatoid arthritis.

7. True: only after articular destruction, capsular stretching and often tendon rupture have occurred do joint instability and deformity follow.

8. False: they are lesions consisting of granulomatous tissue.

9. True: as may the heart, kidney, brain, and gastrointestinal tract.

10. True: although most characteristically they are found under the skin occurring over bony prominences.

11. False: usually rheumatoid arthritis starts as a polyarthritis affecting the small joints of the fingers, wrist, and feet.

12. True: although only 25% of patients with rheumatoid arthritis have rheumatoid nodules.

13. Muscle wasting around deformed joints is rare in rheumatoid arthritis. (1)

14. Characteristically the fingers of a rheumatoid hand deviate in a radial direction. (1)

15. Peripheral neuropathy is not as common in rheumatoid arthritis as in osteoarthritis. (1)

16. Plain lateral and anteroposterior radiographs will exclude cervical instability in rheumatoid patients. (1)

17. Rheumatoid factor is present in 80% of patients with the clinical symptoms of rheumatoid arthritis. (1)

18. High titres of rheumatoid factor and C-reactive protein indicate active disease, but have no predictive value. (1)

19. Polyarthritis must be present for more than 3 months before a diagnosis of rheumatoid arthritis may be considered. (1)

20. Reiter's disease commonly affects the small joints. (1)

21. Rheumatoid factor is also present in systemic lupus erythematosus. (1)

22. In only a minority of patients with rheumatoid arthritis does the disease progress without episodes of remission. (1)

23. Immunosuppressive drugs may be used in aggressive rheumatoid arthritis. (1)

24. Inflammation in joints may be effectively treated by night splinting. (1)

Answers opposite

13. False: often muscle wasting is severe, due to disuse resulting from joint stiffness and pain.

14. False: they deviate in an ulnar direction. In advanced disease subluxation or dislocation of the metacarpophalangeal joints may occur.

15. False: neuropathy occurs in longstanding cases of rheumatoid arthritis reflecting the systemic nature of the disease process.

16. False: in addition to the anteroposterior view, flexion and extension views of the lateral cervical spine should be taken to exclude instability.

17. True

18. False: high titres herald more serious disease.

19. False: involvement of joints for over 6 weeks will satisfy diagnostic criteria.

20. False: it most commonly affects the large joints and the lumbosacral spine. Conjunctivitis and urethritis may also occur.

21. False $\times$ 40% Rh fact posit

22. True: in 80% of patients with rheumatoid arthritis the disease follows a periodic course.

23. True: they have a direct effect on the autoimmune process, but are only administered in severe cases as serious side effects are possible.

24. True: rest is effective, but inflamed joints should be put through a range of passive movement each day to maintain mobility.

25. Ankylosing spondylitis is a chronic inflammatory disorder of spine and sacroiliac joints. (1)

26. In ankylosing spondylitis males are affected 10 times more than females. (1)

27. There is a genetic predisposition to ankylosing spondylitis . What is the particular tissue type associated with the condition?(1)

28. Ankylosing spondylitis may be differentiated from rheumatoid arthritis as symptoms are limited to the sacroiliac joints and spine. (1)

29. What are syndesmophytes?(1)

30. Vertebral osteotomy must be performed early in ankylosing spondylitis to correct deformity and achieve balance to prevent progression. (1)

31. Sacroileitis like that seen in ankylosing spondylitis may also be a feature of Reiter's disease or psoriatic arthritis. (1)

32. 41% of patients have psoriasis on the skin of joints affected by rheumatoid arthritis. This subgroup is classified as 'psoriatic arthritis'. (1)

33. Which joints of the hand does psoriatic arthritis primarily affect?(1)

34. Psoriatic arthropathy may progress to produce arthritis mutilans in the hand. (1)

35. Reiter's disease is a reactive arthritis. (1)

Answers opposite

25. True: patients often present with pain and stiffness of the back.

26. True: they commonly present between 15 and 25 years of age.

27. HLA-B27. This marker is present in 90% of cases.

28. False: approximately 10% of patients with ankylosing spondylitis complain of pain in peripheral joints. These may be swollen or tender.

29. Bony bridges between the vertebral bodies as in ankylosing spondylitis. Bridging at many levels produces a characteristic radiograph appearance of 'bamboo' spine.

30. False: vertebral osteotomy should be reserved for severe cases presenting late with a fixed deformity.

31. True: patients with Reiter's disease and psoriatic arthritis may also show HLA-B27.

32. False: psoriatic arthritis is a different disease entity producing more bone destruction than rheumatoid arthritis.

33. The interphalangeal joints.

34. True: bony destruction may be so aggressive as to produce flail or deformed digits.

35. True: arthritis results from infection in the urogenital or gastrointestinal tracts.

36. In Reiter's disease the organism is carried in the bloodstream from the urogenital tract to the highly vascular large joints to produce an infective arthritis. (1)

37. In Reiter's disease large joint symptoms are present for as long as urogenital or gastrointestinal infection persists. (1)

38. Systemic juvenile chronic arthritis (JCA) may present with fever, rashes, and hepatosplenomegaly. (1).

39. Pauciarticular JCA often produces complications within the eye. (1)

40. What fatal systemic complication may children with longstanding JCA suffer?(1)

41. Joint replacement in children must be delayed until bony maturity and appropriate size are reached. (1)

Total score   41
Target score
    Postgraduate   37
    Undergraduate   30

Answers opposite

36. False: the joints are not infected. The synovium becomes inflamed as a result of the immune response to infection elsewhere.

37. False: 80% of patients continue to have symptoms for many years, long after the urogenital or gastrointestinal infection has settled.

38. True

39. True: 50% of patients suffer chronic iridocyclitis which undetected may lead to blindness.

40. Amyloidosis which arises as a result of long-term chronic inflammation.

41. False: in severe cases, custom built implants may be used.

Gout and Degenerative Arthritis

1. Gout is caused by deposition of urea crystals in joints. (1)

2. Gout is twice as common in men as in women. (1)

3. Myeloproliferative disorders may cause primary gout. (1)

4. Gouty tophi only occur in the ear. (1)

5. Surgery may precipitate an acute attack of gout. (1)

6. Acute gout is always accompanied by hyperuricaemia. (1)

7. The finding of characteristic bifringent crystals in synovial fluid indicates gout. (1)

8. Bridging trabeculae on X-rays are pathognomonic of gout. (1)

9. Allopurinol is the treatment of acute gout. (1)

10. Pseudogout is caused by drinking white wine. (1)

11. Softening of the articular cartilage is the earliest pathological change in primary osteoarthritis. (1)

Answers opposite

Gout and Degenerative Arthritis

1. False: it is due to urate crystal deposition and acute synovitis.

2. False: the figure is closer to 20:1.

3. False: they may cause secondary gout by overproduction of uric acid.

4. False: they may occur around any joint or bursa and in cartilage.

5. True: due to an increase in metabolic breakdown products.

6. False: the level may fluctuate although it is generally raised.

7. True

8. False: during an acute attack of gout there may be soft tissue swelling seen on X-ray. Chronic gout may reveal juxta-articular 'punched out' cysts, joint space narrowing and secondary osteoarthritic changes.

9. False: this may cause a temporary flare up of the gout. A non-steroidal anti-inflammatory drug, e.g. indomethacin, should be given and once the acute attack has settled, allopurinol or probenecid may be considered.

10. False: it is caused by deposition of calcium pyrophosphate dihydrate in joint tissues.

11. True: this then becomes frayed or fibrillated and is worn away.

12. Give four causes of secondary osteoarthritis. (4)

13. What are the characteristic radiological features of osteoarthritis?(4)

14. Physiotherapy is of no benefit in the treatment of osteoarthritis. (1)

15. Charcot joints are usually painful. (1)

16. Charcot joints are commonly caused by herpes. (1)

17. Haemophilia seldom affects joints. (1)

18. Heberden's nodes in osteoarthritis occur most commonly in men. (1)

Total score	24
Target score	
Postgraduate	21
Undergraduate	18

Answers opposite

Gout and Degenerative Arthritis

- Congenital (Developmental) → Congenital hip dislocation
- Metabolic → CPPD
- Trauma eg fracture, surgery, Repetitive use.
- Inflammatory → RA, SA, Gout.

12. Any four from:
Previous trauma to the articular surface
Previous infection
Inflammatory arthritis, e.g. rheumatoid arthritis
Joint deformity
Excessive stresses, e.g. overweight

13. Narrowing of the joint space, periarticular sclerosis, bone cysts, osteophytes.

14. False: it is of significant benefit in symptom relief, especially in osteoarthritis of the knees.

15. False: it is because the protective reflexes stimulated by pain are not present that the articular destruction seen in Charcot joints occurs.

ic Tabes dorsalis
16. False: syphilitic neuropathy is one cause, others are peripheral neuropathies (acquired and congenital), cauda equina lesions and syringomyelia.

17. False: repeated bleeding into joints causes chronic synovitis which may be followed by cartilage degeneration.

18. False: they are more common in postmenopausal women.

Bone Necrosis

1. Gaucher's disease is commonest in people from South East Asia. (1)

2. Give three clinical disorders which may be associated with osteonecrosis. (3)

3. Articular cartilage overlying areas of osteonecrosis rapidly shows degenerative changes. (1)

4. Radionuclide scanning is diagnostic in osteonecrosis. (1)

5. Give three sites where avascular necrosis may follow fracture or dislocation. (3)

6. Sickle cell disease affects people of Central and West African descent. (1)

7. In sickle cell disease hypoxia may precipitate bone crises with clumping of sickle-shaped cells in bone capillaries. (1)

8. In sickle cell disease, infarction of structures other than bone rarely occurs. (1)

9. Release of nitrogen from the blood and fat causes osteonecrosis in decompression sickness (caisson disease). (1)

10. Gaucher's disease has a viral aetiology. (1)

Answers opposite

Bone Necrosis

1. False: it occurs predominantly in Ashkenazy Jews.

2. Any three of:
   Trauma
   Perthes' disease
   Sickle cell disease
   Caisson disease
   Gaucher's disease
   Alcohol abuse
   Any disease requiring steroid therapy

3. False: the cartilage is nourished by synovial fluid thus it is preserved until late in osteonecrosis when collapse of the underlying bone causes fragmentation of the articular surface.

4. False: the result usually shows a 'cold' area over the section of dead bone, but results may be confused by 'hot' areas due to a vascular reaction in the area of the surrounding bone.

5. The three most common: femoral head, carpal bones (e.g. scaphoid and lunate), talus.

6. True: due to an inherited disorder in haemoglobin.

7. True: if severe, bone infarction and osteonecrosis may follow.

8. False: infarction commonly occurs in the lungs or kidneys. Patients may also present with acute abdominal crises after infarction of the intestine.

9. True: tissues become supersaturated with nitrogen under pressure which is released as bubbles during rapid decompression. The nitrogen bubbles then occlude the capillaries to the bone.

10. False: it is a familial disorder, producing an abnormal accumulation of glucocerebroside.

11. Unlike sickle cell disease, Gaucher deposits do not get infected. (1)

12. Characteristic X-ray changes in Gaucher's disease include expansion of the tubular bones. (1)

13. The femoral and humeral heads and femoral condyles are common sites of osteonecrosis caused by corticosteroids and alcohol abuse. (1)

14. Which two of the following conditions are due to osteochondritis: Kienbock's disease, clergyman's knee, spondylolisthesis, Panner's disease? (2)

15. Osteochondritis dissecans results from minor trauma causing an osteochondral fracture. (1)

16. The base of the 1st metacarpal is a common site for osteochondritis dissecans. (1)

17. Osgood Schlatter's disease and Sever's disease are both caused by the same mechanism. (1)

Total score	22
Target score	
Postgraduate	20
Undergraduate	17

Answers opposite

11. False: similar to infection of bone infarcts in sickle cell disease, patients with Gaucher's may present with septicaemia.

12. True: most particularly the distal femur producing the Erlen–Meyer flask appearance.

13. True: probably caused by fatty changes within the marrow and subsequent infarction.

14. Kienbock's disease of the lunate and Panner's disease of the capitulum are both due to osteochondritis.

15. True: large osteochondral fragments may be pinned back in position. Small fragments causing symptoms of pain or locking are usually removed.

16. False: the most common sites are the medial femoral condyle, the talus and the capitulum.

17. True: respectively at the unfused apophysis of the tibial tubercle and calcaneum, they are caused by the traction of the attached tendon.

Metabolic and Endocrine Disorders

1. Vitamin D can only be obtained from dietary sources. (1)

2. In which two organs is vitamin D (cholecalciferol) activated?(2)

3. Vitamin D stimulates the uptake of calcium by the small intestine. (1)

4. Parathyroid hormone causes a lowering of serum calcium. (1)

5. In rickets there is inadequate mineralization of growing bone. (1)

6. The bony deformity in rickets only affects the limbs. (1)

7. The X-ray appearances in rickets show cupped metaphyses. (1)

8. Rickets only occurs in vitamin D deficiency. (1)

9. In rickets the alkaline phosphatase level is raised. (1)

Mildly ↓ Ca²⁺ , Po⁴ ↓ , alk phos ↑ , vit D↓ , PTH ↑

10. In osteomalacia, like rickets, there is inadequate mineralization of bone. (1)

11. Pathological fractures are rare in osteomalacia. (1)

Answers opposite

Metabolic and Endocrine Disorders

1. False: it can be synthesized by the action of ultraviolet light on precursors in the skin.

2. In the liver to form 25-hydroxycholecalciferol and then in the kidney to give 1,25-dihydroxycholecalciferol.

3. True

4. False: it causes an increase by increasing osteoclastic bone resorption, increasing tubular reabsorption of calcium, and increasing production of 1,25-dihydroxycholecalciferol (active vitamin D).

5. True

6. False: there may also be deformity in the skull (craniotabes), enlargement of the costochondral junctions and lateral indentation of the chest (Harrison's sulcus). There may also be vertebral and pelvic deformities.

7. True

8. False: it may also occur in hypophosphataemia due to genetic causes (familial hypophosphataemia) or due to impaired renal tubular reabsorption of phosphate (renal tubular rickets).

9. True

10. True

11. False: the weakened bone breaks easily and heals poorly.

12. Radiological appearances in osteomalacia are usually normal. (1)

13. Biochemical changes are often insignificant in osteomalacia. (1)

14. Osteomalacia may occur secondary to liver disorders. (1)

15. Primary hyperparathyroidism is usually due to a benign adenoma. (1)

16. In secondary hyperparathyroidism the serum calcium is usually raised. (1)

17. List four clinical features of hyperparathyroidism. (4)

18. What radiological sign is diagnostic of hyperparathyroidism?(1)

19. Scurvy is caused by a deficiency of vitamin B. (1)

20. The underlying pathology in scurvy is failure of maturation of collagen. (1)

21. Scurvy may present in children as pseudoparalysis. (1)

Answers opposite

12. False: there is generalized rarefaction and there may be signs of old fractures. 'Looser zones' may be present. These are transverse radiolucent bands around poorly healing stress fractures. There may also be subperiosteal resorption due to secondary hyperparathyroidism.

13. True: diagnosis is often made on bone biopsy demonstrating excessive unmineralized osteoid.

14. True: liver disease may affect the availability of 25-dihydroxycholecalciferol.

15. True

16. False: it is commonly low, indeed it is the hypocalcaemia that stimulates the secondary hyperparathyroidism.

17. Any four from:
    Anorexia
    Nausea
    Depression
    Abdominal pain
    Polyuria
    Urinary tract infections
    Bony pain
    Pathological fracture

18. Subperiosteal bone resorption. This is best seen in a plain film of the hand.

19. False: it is caused by a deficiency of vitamin C (ascorbic acid).

20. True

21. True: subperiosteal haemorrhage may cause such severe pain that the child refuses to use the limb.

22. In scurvy there is an increased tendency to tooth decay. (1)

23. Bone mass in men seldom decreases with age. (1)

24. List three sites where pathological fractures commonly occur in osteoporosis. (3)

25. Fluoride may be used to treat osteoporosis. (1)

26. Regular exercise helps prevent osteoporosis. (1)

27. Paget's disease is more common in men than women. (1)

28. In Paget's disease bones are thicker and stronger than normal. (1)

29. Paget's disease characteristically causes bowing of the legs. (1)

30. In Paget's disease, serum acid phosphatase is usually raised. (1)

31. Paget's disease may turn malignant. (1)

32. There is increased risk of slipped upper femoral epiphysis in both hypopituitary dwarfism and hyperpituitary gigantism. (1)

33. Hyperthyroidism produces marble bone disease (osteopetrosis). (1)

Total score 39
Target score
    Postgraduate 36
    Undergraduate 30

Answers opposite

22. False: the gums however are spongy and minor trauma may cause bleeding.

23. False: senile osteoporosis occurs in both sexes but in women the decrease in bone mass is more marked and more rapid after the menopause.

24. Vertebrae – crush fractures
    Femoral neck
    Distal radius

25. True

26. True

27. False: it affects both men and women equally.

28. False: there are alternating phases of rapid bone formation and destruction resulting in a thickened but irregular cortex which is weaker than normal and prone to pathological fractures.

29. True: it was originally termed 'osteitis deformans'.

30. False: alkaline phosphatase is usually raised because of rapid turnover of bone.

31. True: in approximately 1% of cases malignant change can occur resulting in osteosarcoma. This is more common in the elderly and has a very poor prognosis.

32. True: this is because both the above are associated with sexual immaturity and delayed closure of epiphyses.

33. False: the aetiology of osteopetrosis is unclear.

Bone Dysplasias

1. Patients with bone dysplasias who measure below 1.5 metres in height are classified as dwarfs. (1)

2. Patients with Hurler's disease are proportionate dwarfs. (1)

3. Achondroplasia is an inherited disorder only. (1)

4. Type 2 osteogenesis imperfecta is inherited as an autosomal dominant condition. (1)

5. Blue sclerae are found in type 4 osteogenesis imperfecta. (1)

6. Osteogenesis imperfecta may be fatal. (1)

7. In hereditary multiple exostoses (diaphyseal aclasis), bony exostoses occur at the metaphyses as the bone grows. (1)

8. Because of the risk of malignant change to chondrosarcoma, exostoses should be removed early. (1)

9. Dyschondroplasia (Ollier's disease) is typically unilateral. (1)

10. In Ollier's disease the affected limbs are short. (1)

11. Correction of deformity in Ollier's disease should be carried out early to arrest progression of the deformity. (1)

12. Multiple epiphyseal dysplasia affects the epiphyses to cause bony overgrowth and taller than average patients. (1)

Answers opposite

Bone Dysplasias

1. False: patients must be less than 1.25 metres in height to be classified as dwarfs.

2. True: this rare monopolysaccharide disorder produces dwarfing of both trunk and legs.

3. False: the disorder may be inherited as an autosomal dominant condition, but the majority of cases occur sporadically.

4. False: some variants (type 1) are autosomal dominant, others are sporadic or autosomal recessive (types 2 and 3).

5. False: blue sclerae are found in type 1 (the commonest) but not in type 4.

6. True: in the severe type 2 multiple fractures occur *in utero* or at birth and the infant may not survive.

7. True

8. False: only a tiny minority of exostoses develop chondrosarcomatous change. Only an exostosis that continues to grow after bony maturity has been reached should be removed to exclude malignant change.

9. True

10. True

11. False: early correction will be lost as the disorder in the epiphyseal plate will cause the deformity to recur. Corrective osteotomy should be delayed until bony maturity.

12. False: this disorder produces shorter patients.

13. What is arachnodactyly?(1)

14. Patients with Marfan's syndrome suffer cardiovascular complications. (1)

15. Patients with Marfan's syndrome develop scoliosis, but have no vertebral anomalies. (1)

16. Marfan's disorder is inherited as an autosomal recessive condition. (1)

17. Neurofibromatosis is associated with generalized joint laxity. (1)

18. Neurofibromatosis may cause compression of nerve roots due to tumours in the spinal canal. (1)

19. Café au lait spots over the spine in neurofibromatosis indicate a tendency to develop scoliosis in later life. (1)

20. Cystic ares in fibrous dysplasia do not occur in the epiphyses. (1)

21. Patients with fibrous dysplasia may present with a pathological fracture. (1)

22. Albright's disease is fibrous dysplasia in association with delayed puberty. (1)

Total	22
Target score	
Postgraduate	20
Undergraduate	15

Answers opposite

13. Long, thin fingers (spider fingers).

14. True: due to a defect in collagen formation, they suffer aortic aneurysms.

15. True

16. False: autosomal dominant.

17. False: joint laxity classically occurs with Marfan's syndrome.

18. True

19. False: there is no association.

20. True: they occur mainly in the diaphyses or metaphyses.

21. True: fibrous replacement of sections of bone leads to weakening and possibly fracture.

22. False: puberty is precocious.

Tumours

1. Primary bone tumours are more common than secondary metastatic deposits in bone. (1)

2. Malignant bone tumours can usually be diagnosed clinically. (1)

3. The osteoid osteoma causes pain which is characteristically relieved by rest. (1)

4. The radiological features of an osteoid osteoma consist of an area of dense sclerosis with a small central radiolucent spot. (1)

5. The osteochondroma is the most common malignant tumour of bone. (1)

6. X-ray appearances underestimate the size of osteochondromata. (1)

7. The condition of multiple osteochondromata is known as Ollier's disease. (1)

8. Chrondromata may turn malignant. (1)

9. Solitary bone cysts as incidental X-ray findings become more rare as age increases. (1)

10. Solitary bone cysts can be treated with injection of corticosteroids. (1)

11. Aneurysmal bone cysts are usually confined to the metaphyseal side of the growth plate. (1)

12. Fibrous cortical defects are usually treated by curettage and bone grafting. (1)

Answers opposite

Tumours

1. False: metastatic deposits are much more common especially in the over 50s.

2. False: definitive diagnosis usually requires radiographic imaging and biopsy.

3. False: the pain is usually unrelieved by rest but often responds to aspirin.

4. True: the radiolucent centre is known as a nidus.

5. False: it is the most common tumour but it is usually benign.

6. True: because there is often a radiolucent cartilage cap.

7. False: it is known as diaphyseal aclasia. Ollier's disease is multiple enchondromata.

8. True: especially in patients over 30 and in large bones.

9. True: it is therefore presumed that many disappear spontaneously.

10. True: they also often disappear after fracture through the cyst wall.

11. True: giant cell tumours on the other hand, which may resemble aneurysmal bone cysts radiologically, may extend to the articular surface.

12. False: the majority require no treatment.

13. Giant cell tumours are nearly always benign. (1)

14. Giant cell tumours usually occur between the ages of 20 and 40. (1)

15. Osteosarcoma usually only spreads locally. (1)

16. Osteosarcoma is more common in the elderly. (1)

17. Sunray spicules are characteristic X-ray findings in chondrosarcoma. (1)

18. Osteosarcoma is commonly found in the proximal femur and distal tibia. (1)

19. Ewing's tumour is a malignant proliferation of osteocytes. (1)

20. Ewing's tumour occurs mainly in the elderly. (1)

21. What characteristic X-ray changes are often seen in Ewing's tumour?(1)

22. Multiple myeloma commonly presents with back pain. (1)

23. Name two investigations used in myeloma. (2)

24. The majority of metastatic bony tumours arise from carcinoma of the breast or prostate. (1)

Answers opposite

13. False

14. True

15. False: it is often highly malignant and metastasises widely, especially to the lungs.

16. False: the incidence is highest at between 10 and 20, but there is a second and smaller peak after the age of 50 because of malignant change in Paget's disease.

17. False: they are commonly seen in osteosarcoma.

18. False: it is the opposite. The tumour is commonly found around the knee, in the distal femur and proximal tibia.

19. False: it is a malignant tumour of vascular endothelium.

20. False: it commonly occurs between the ages of 10 and 20.

21. 'Onion skin' layers. These consist of new bone laid down by the raised periosteum.

22. True

23. Any of:
Raised erythrocyte sedimentation rate
Bence Jones' protein in urine
Plasma electrophoresis
Sternal marrow puncture

24. True: other carcinomas commonly metastasizing to bone are thyroid, kidney, lung, and bowel.

25. Pathological fractures of long bones usually heal well with conservative management. (1)

26. Metastatic bone tumours commonly cause hypocalcaemia. (1)

27. Pathological fractures can be caused by minimal forces. (1)

Total score   28
Target score
     Postgraduate   25
     Undergraduate   20

Answers opposite

25. False: they seldom heal well and often require internal fixation.

26. False: hypercalcaemia is often seen. This may require medical treatment.

27. True: even getting out of bed can cause fracture through a metastatic lesion.

Neuromuscular Disorders

1. A flaccid paresis results from a lower motor neuron lesion. (1)

2. Serum creatine phosphokinase is raised in muscular dystrophies. (1)

3. Electromyography does not allow differentiation between polio and weakness due to a muscular dystrophy. (1)

4. Joint deformity follows balanced paralysis of the muscles acting upon it. (1)

5. Unilateral balanced paralysis in a child with equal limb lengths may result in later limb shortening. (1)

6. Cerebral palsy may progressively involve the upper limbs if the lower limbs are primarily involved. (1)

7. Children with cerebral palsy may exhibit both muscular weakness and spasticity. (1)

8. Motor and sensory abilities are only affected in cerebral palsy. Mental function remains normal. (1)

9. Hip flexion and adduction deformities in cerebral palsy give rise to a 'scissoring' gait. (1)

10. Because of abnormal muscle tensions in cerebral palsy, operative procedures should be directed at bony correction of joint deformities. (1)

11. Following a stroke in an adult, physiotherapy is delayed until muscle power has returned and reached grade 2, to allow proper participation in exercises. (1)

Answers opposite

Neuromuscular Disorders

1. True: an upper motor neuron lesion causes spastic paresis.

2. True

3. False: it is of diagnostic value distinguishing between neurological and muscle disease.

4. False: the limb may become floppy or flail, but has no deforming forces acting upon it.

5. True: paralysed limbs fail to grow normally.

6. False: by definition, cerebral palsy is a non-progressive disorder.

7. True

8. False: mental retardation may be present.

9. True: physiotherapy and retraining may be required.

10. False: it the joints are mobile, they may be corrected by re-routing or dividing muscles or tendons. Bony correction is seldom necessary.

11. False: early, daily passive physiotherapy is vital to prevent joint contractures.

12. Meningocele implies herniation of dural sac but not the spinal cord through the defect of spina bifida. (1)

13. Spina bifida usually occurs in the lumbar region. (1)

14. Beta-2 microglobulin in amniotic fluid indicates the presence of spina bifida in the fetus. (1)

15. In babies with open spina bifida, hydrocephalus is common. (1)

16. The anterior horn cells are damaged by virus in poliomyelitis. (1)

17. Following the initial paralysis of poliomyelitis the level of disability remains constant. (1)

18. Polio affects the limb muscles. Trunk muscles are left intact. (1)

19. Poliomyelitis produces an unbalanced paralysis which results in flail joints. (1)

20. Duchenne muscular dystrophy is an autosomal dominant inheritance. (1)

21. Peroneal muscular atrophy (Charcot–Marie–Tooth disease) only affects the peripheral nerves supplying the lower limb. (1)

22. Friedreich's ataxia is an inherited disorder affecting the cerebellum and posterolateral columns of the spinal cord. (1)

Total	22
Target score	
Postgraduate	19
Undergraduate	15

Answers opposite

12. True: meningomyelocele implies both dural and spinal cord herniation.

13. True: incidence of 3 in 1000 overall.

14. False: alphafetoprotein is the indicator of spina bifida *in utero*.

15. True: due to the obstruction of the normal flow of cerebrospinal fluid.

16. True: this gives rise to the characteristic motor paralysis, with normal sensation.

17. False: some anterior horn cells have not been damaged by the virus, but suffer temporary disorder due to oedema. Recovery in these cells may take place over the following two years.

18. False: paralysis of trunk muscles may result in a scoliosis.

19. False: it may produce an unbalanced paralysis which results in deformity, or a balanced paralysis which gives a flail joint.

20. False: it is sex-linked recessive only affecting boys.

21. False: the peripheral nerves and spinal cord are affected throughout, often producing a claw hand in addition to pes cavus foot deformities.

22. True: patients present with clumsiness and ataxia.

Peripheral Nerve Lesions

1. Neurapraxia results in permanent loss of nerve function. (1)

2. Axonotmesis means axonal separation. (1)

3. Axonal regeneration proceeds at the rate of approximately 2.5 cm per month. (1)

4. Denervated skin is smooth, dry and shiny. (1)

5. Nerve repair is best performed under tension. (1)

6. Erb's palsy refers to a lesion of the lower trunks of the brachial plexus. (1)

7. Where nerve roots have been avulsed from the spinal cord recovery is impossible. (1)

8. Birth injuries to the brachial plexus should be treated with splintage of the arm while awaiting recovery. (1)

9. Axillary nerve injuries following shoulder dislocation seldom recover. (1)

10. Following an isolated radial nerve injury the patient is unable to straighten the fingers. (1)

Answers opposite

Peripheral Nerve Lesions

1. False: in neurapraxia the axons remain intact and there is spontaneous recovery of function, usually within a few weeks.

2. True: although the axons are disrupted the investing connective tissue sheaths are intact thus the regenerating axon can be guided to its correct destination.

3. True: about 2.5 cm per month or 1 mm a day.

4. True: denervation results in trophic changes and there is also loss of autonomic function.

5. False: if it is not possible to perform primary repair without tension, a nerve graft should be used.

6. False: it is an injury to the upper part of the plexus (C5 and C6) resulting in paralysis of shoulder abductors and external rotators. Sensation is lost along the outer aspect of the arm. Klumpke's palsy describes an injury to the lower trunks of the brachial plexus.

7. True

8. False: the mother should maintain passive movements to prevent fixed deformities.

9. False: spontaneous recovery is usual.

10. False: the fingers can be straightened using the intrinsic muscles (supplied by median and ulnar nerves), but cannot be extended at the metacarpophalangeal joints since the long finger extensors are supplied by the radial nerve.

11. Radial nerve injuries result in sensory loss over the entire dorsum of the hand. (1)

12. The ulnar nerve is very susceptible to damage by wounds on the lateral side of the elbow. (1)

13. Lesions of the ulnar nerve cause clawing of the fingers due to weakness of the extensor muscles of the forearm. (1)

14. Gaps in the ulnar nerve following injury can be approximated by transposing the nerve to the front of the elbow. (1)

15. Division of the median nerve causes loss of sensation to the medial three and a half digits. (1)

16. Division of the radial nerve at the wrist causes significant motor weakness of the hand. (1)

17. Following median nerve injury, abduction and opposition of the thumb are weak. (1)

18. Lesions of the lumbosacral plexus complicating sacral fractures are treated by early exploration. (1)

19. Pressure on L3 and L4 nerve roots causes weakness of knee extension and a decreased knee jerk. (1)

20. Pressure on L5 nerve root by a prolapsed intervertebral disc causes weakness of big toe plantar flexion. (1)

21. Pressure on S1 causes a weak ankle jerk. (1)

Answers opposite

11. False: the radial nerve supplies sensation to the back of the hand. However there is considerable overlap of supply by the median and ulnar nerves so the resultant sensory loss is usually only noticeable over the dorsum of the first web space.

12. False: the nerve runs on the medial side of the elbow although it should be checked for damage in any wound around the elbow.

13. False: the clawing is due to paralysis of the intrinsic muscles (the lumbricals and interossei).

14. True: this effectively shortens the course of the ulnar nerve.

15. False: sensation is lost over the palmar aspect of the radial or lateral three and a half digits.

16. False: Below the wrist the radial nerve is purely sensory.

17. True: the only muscle in the thenar eminence not supplied by the median nerve is the adductor pollicis, which is supplied by the ulnar nerve.

18. False: recovery is usually quite good and exploration is seldom helpful.

19. True: there is also a loss of sensation over the anterior thigh and medial side of the leg.

20. False: it causes weakness of big toe extension and decreased sensation over the front and lateral side of the leg and the medial border of the foot.

21. True: there is also weak ankle plantar flexion and decreased sensation on the lateral border and sole of the foot.

22. Sphincter disturbance following prolapsed intervertebral disc is best treated by bed rest and physiotherapy. (1)

23. Femoral nerve injuries are common following hip dislocation. (1)

24. Pressure from a below-knee plaster may damage the lateral popliteal nerve. (1)

25. Pregnancy causes relaxation of ligaments and usually relieves symptoms of carpal tunnel syndrome. (1)

26. Sudeck's atrophy of the hand may follow myocardial infarction. (1)

Total score   26
Target score
    Postgraduate   24
    Undergraduate   22

Answers opposite

22. False: this is a sign of sacral root pressure and is an indication for urgent surgery to explore and decompress the cauda equina.

23. False: the sciatic nerve is much more likely to be damaged by traction or by direct pressure from a posterior dislocation.

24. True: this nerve winds around the neck of the fibula and is prone to damage by local pressure or varus deformity of the knee.

25. False: there is usually increased fluid retention in pregnancy and carpal tunnel syndrome is often exacerbated.

26. True: although the most common cause is a local injury to the upper limb.

Orthopaedic Operations

1. What two permanent complications may arise from leaving a tourniquet on too long?(2)

2. Tourniquets should be inflated by 100 mmHg above the diastolic blood pressure to provide a bloodless field. (1)

3. Allografts (homografts) are bone grafts which come from a different part of the same body. (1)

4. Unlike other organs, bone grafts taken from cadavers do not need to be screened for HIV. (1)

5. Leg length inequality up to 2.5 cm does not usually require surgical treatment. (1)

6. Trauma is the cause of most limb amputations in the UK. (1)

7. In an above-knee amputation the weight of the body is transferred through the ischial tuberosity on to the prosthesis. (1)

8. What microbe causes gas gangrene?(1)

9. Gas gangrene is commoner in below-knee than in above-knee amputations. (1)

10. Phantom-limb sensation is the feeling that the amputated limb is still present. This usually disappears. (1)

Total	11
Target score	
Postgraduate	10
Undergraduate	8

Answers opposite

Orthopaedic Operations

1. Nerve damage – due to pressure. Muscle necrosis and contracture due to ischaemia.

2. False: 100 mmHg above the *systolic* pressure.

3. False: they come from a different individual of the same species.

4. False: all tissues should be checked.

5. True: above 2.5 cm, treatment should be considered.

6. False: peripheral vascular disease is the cause of most amputations.

7. True: the amputation stump should not be weight bearing.

8. Clostridia.

9. False: clostridia spores from the perineum contaminate the wound. Thus infection of the above-knee amputation is more likely.

10. True

The Shoulder

1. Pain in myocardial infarction may be referred to the tip of the shoulder. (1)

2. The shoulder should be examined from the front. (1)

3. With anterior dislocation the shoulder is held in internal rotation. (1)

4. Pain in the midrange of abduction suggests a rotator cuff lesion. (1)

5. Reaching up the back with the fingers tests internal rotation of the shoulder. (1)

6. When the glenohumeral joint is fused, no abduction of the shoulder is possible. (1)

7. Damage to the nerve supply of the latissimus dorsi muscle results in winging of the scapula. (1)

8. Pectoralis major is tested by asking the patient to push both hands into the waist. (1)

9. An anteroposterior X-ray of the shoulder is sufficient. (1)

10. The scapulae develop in the neck and descend to the thorax by the third month of fetal life. (1)

11. Acromioclavicular subluxation seldom needs surgical fixation. (1)

12. The rotator cuff comprises the subscapularis, supraspinatus, infraspinatus and teres major muscles. (1)

Answers opposite

The Shoulder

1. True

2. False: the shoulder should be examined from both the front and the back.

3. False: internal rotation occurs with posterior dislocation.

4. True

5. True

6. False: scapulothoracic movement allows up to 90° of abduction.

7. False: winging of the scapula is caused by paralysis of the serratus anterior supplied by the long thoracic nerve (C5/6/7).

8. True

9. False: at least two views should be obtained, e.g. an anteroposterior and an axillary projection.

10. True: bilateral failure of scapula descent associated with cervical vertebral anomalies is known as Klippel–Feil syndrome.

11. True: shoulder function is rarely compromised.

12. False: the first three are correct but it is teres *minor* not major.

13. Autopsy studies show that most patients over 60 have small tears of the rotator cuff. (1)

14. The commonest site of rotator cuff tears is the subscapularis. (1)

15. Rotator cuff injuries are usually more painful in younger than older patients. (1)

16. Deposits of calcium hydroxyapatite in the supraspinatus tendon occur mainly in chronic tendinitis. (1)

17. Acute calcific tendinitis may be helped by surgical removal of the calcific material. (1)

18. Chronic supraspinatus tendinitis usually gives a painful arc at between 0° and 60° of abduction. (1)

19. Surgical excision of the coracoacromial ligament and part of the acromion may be necessary if conservative treatment of the painful arc syndrome is not successful. (1)

20. Frozen shoulder is uncommon in the under 60s. (1)

21. In frozen shoulder the normal course of events is initial stiffness followed by pain. (1)

22. Arthrography in frozen shoulder reveals a stretched joint capsule. (1)

23. Shoulder stiffness may follow a cerebrovascular accident. (1)

24. Rotator cuff tears result in immediate pain and inability to initiate abduction of the arm. (1)

Answers opposite

13. True: these are often asymptomatic.

14. False: the most common site of injury is the 'critical zone' of the supraspinatus. This is a relatively avascular area near its insertion.

15. True

16. False: this phenomenon whose cause is unknown occurs in acute supraspinatus tendinitis. It is usually accompanied by severe pain due to local swelling.

17. True: pain relief follows decompression.

18. False: the painful arc is usually at 60–120° because it is at this degree of abduction that the injured and congested area of the tendon passes under the confined area of the coracoacromial arch.

19. True

20. False: it is most common in the 40–60 age group.

21. False: usually the first symptom is pain and as this subsides the shoulder becomes more stiff. The stiffness may persist for 6–12 months before slowly improving.

22. False: the capsule is contracted.

23. True because of inactivity and muscle spasm.

24. True

25. Complete rotator cuff tears usually regain full function with conservative management. (1)

26. Contrast arthrography of the shoulder joint may be used to demonstrate rotator cuff tears. (1)

27. Rupture of the long head of biceps usually requires surgical repair. (1)

28. X-ray of a case of tuberculosis of the shoulder is likely to show a dense sclerotic reaction. (1)

29. The shoulder is seldom involved in rheumatoid disease. (1)

30. Chronic synovitis of the shoulder may lead to rupture of the rotator cuff and joint erosion. (1)

31. Osteoarthritis of the shoulder is usually secondary to other pathology. (1)

Total score	31
Target score	
Postgraduate	29
Undergraduate	25

Answers opposite

25. False: in younger patients these should be repaired surgically.

26. True: arthroscopy may also be used.

27. False: once the initial pain has settled, good function usually returns despite a change in shape of the biceps muscle.

28. False: generalized rarefaction is present and there may be erosion of the joint surfaces.

29. False: this joint is frequently involved.

30. True: these changes occur in rheumatoid arthritis.

31. True

The Elbow

1. Pain from the elbow joint is commonly localized to the condyles. (1)

2. Pathological processes in the elbow may give rise to weakness and tingling in the hand. (1)

3. Golfer's elbow is painful medial epicondylitis. (1)

4. 'Gun stock' deformity may follow a supracondylar fracture. (1)

5. In tennis elbow examination often reveals a small fluid-filled cyst over the lateral epicondyle. (1)

6. The majority of tennis elbows require a local steroid injection to ameliorate symptoms. (1)

7. The close congruity of the joint surfaces of the elbow mean that in cases of tuberculosisB of the elbow, surgical debridement and excision of the joint surfaces are necessary. (1)

8. The elbow is involved in approximately 50% of patients with rheumatoid arthritis. (1)

Answers opposite

The Elbow

1. False: pain from the joint itself is diffusely spread.

2. True: due to the close proximity of the ulnar nerve to the elbow joint.

3. True: tennis elbow is lateral epicondylitis.

4. True: gunstock deformity is cubitus varus which may follow malunion of a supracondylar fracture.

5. False: but there is usually tenderness just below the lateral epicondyle.

6. False: most heal spontaneously if rested.

7. False: antituberculous chemotherapy is often all that is required. Surgical debridement of the synovium only is very rarely needed.

8. True

9. Unlike the knee, loose bodies within the elbow joint rarely cause locking. (1)

10. Calcification in olecranon bursa is indicative of chronic infection. (1)

11. Ulnar nerve symptoms following malunion of a supracondylar fracture may arise many months after the union of bone has occurred. (1)

Total   11
Target score
    Postgraduate   9
    Undergraduate   8

Answers opposite

9. False: loose bodies cause symptomatic locking and should be removed.

10. False: the most likely cause of calcification in an olecranon bursa is gout.

11. True: this is tardy ulnar palsy. The treatment is to transpose the ulnar nerve to the front of the elbow.

The Wrist

1. Stiffness and deformity in the wrist are usually noticed early by the patient. (1)

2. Examination of the wrist is not complete without examination of elbow, forearm and hand. (1)

3. Pain in the wrist is often localized to either side or to the dorsum. (1)

4. The scaphoid bone is best seen with anteroposterior and lateral wrist X-rays. (1)

5. Radial club hand is a rare deformity involving overgrowth of the radius. (1)

6. In Madelung's deformity the wrist is deviated to the ulnar side. (1)

7. De Quervain's disease is due to stenosing tenovaginitis of the extensor pollicis longus tendon. (1)

8. De Quervain's disease is commonest in men. (1)

9. Adduction of the wrist with the thumb enclosed in a clenched fist causes severe pain in cases of De Quervain's disease. (1)

10. Ununited scaphoid fractures are characteristically tender over the anterior aspect of the bone. (1)

11. X-rays of avascular necrosis of the scaphoid usually show decreased density in the avascular fragment. (1)

12. Osteoarthritis of the metacarpophalangeal joint of the thumb is common. (1)

Answers opposite

The Wrist

1. False: they are both often late symptoms.

2. True

3. True

4. False: special oblique views of the scaphoid are necessary to show up difficult fractures.

5. False: in this congenital condition the radius is absent and the wrist is deviated to the radial side.

6. True

7. False: it is due to stenosing tenovaginitis but the tendons involved are the extensor pollicis brevis and abductor pollicis longus.

8. False: it is most common in women aged 30–50.

9. True: this is the basis of Finkelstein's test.

10. False: it is the anatomical snuff box that is usually the site of most tenderness.

11. False: avascular necrosis usually causes increased density.

12. False: it is the carpometacarpal joint of the thumb that more commonly shows osteoarthritic changes.

13. Kienbock's disease describes avascular necrosis of the second metacarpal. (1)

14. A short ulna may be associated with Kienbock's disease. (1)

15. Tuberculosis of the wrist usually presents late as an established arthritis. (1)

16. Tuberculosis of the wrist is usually bilateral. (1)

17. Both tuberculous and rheumatoid arthritis can cause extensive carpal destruction. (1)

18. Synovitis of the wrist in rheumatoid arthritis often causes erosion and rupture of flexor tendons. (1)

19. Wrist arthrodesis or arthroplasty is best performed in the early stages of rheumatoid arthritis. (1)

20. Osteoarthritis of the wrist usually only occurs as a sequel to trauma or inflammatory arthritis. (1)

21. Ganglia on the dorsum of the wrist are associated with an underlying vascular abnormality. (1)

22. Ganglia are usually treated by hitting them with the family Bible. (1)

23. Carpal tunnel syndrome is commonest in male labourers. (1)

Answers opposite

13. False: it is avascular necrosis of the lunate. The pathogenesis is not fully understood but it may follow acute or chronic trauma.

14. True: this is called negative ulnar variance. The prominent corner of the distal radius may cause repetitive trauma to the lunate and predispose to Kienbock's disease.

15. True

16. False: bilateral chronic arthritis of the wrist is nearly always rheumatoid in origin.

17. True

18. False: it more commonly causes rupture of extensor tendons.

19. False: these procedures are indicated late in the disease after joint destruction has occurred.

20. True

21. False

22. False: although this method may undoubtedly work; aspiration or multiple puncture as an outpatient procedure is more usual, followed by excision if the ganglion recurs. Many ganglia are asymptomatic and are therefore best left alone.

23. False: it is most common in women, especially during pregnancy and after the menopause.

24. In carpal tunnel syndrome electrical studies show slowing of conduction of the median nerve across the wrist. (1)

25. Symptoms of carpal tunnel are worse when the wrist is being used. (1)

26. Holding the affected wrist in flexion for 1 minute may reproduce the symptoms of carpal tunnel syndrome. (1).

27. Carpal tunnel syndrome is usually treated by surgical division of the flexor retinaculum. (1)

Total score 27
Target score
        Postgraduate 25
        Undergraduate 20

Answers opposite

24. True: this is true for most cases, however there are some cases where conduction is normal but symptoms are still relieved by division of the flexor retinaculum.

25. False: they are most common at night or when the wrist is kept immobile, e.g. holding a newspaper.

26. True: this is the basis of Phalen's test. The other commonly used clinical test is Tinel's in which tapping over the carpal tunnel causes tingling in the thumb and radial two and a half fingers.

27. True: local steroid injection is sometimes used but its effects are often only temporary.

The Hand

1. Stereognosis is the ability to differentiate between two objects held in the right and left hand. (1)

2. Syndactyly is the joining together of fingers due to a failure of differentiation. (1)

3. Dupuytren's contracture is a thickening of the fibrous flexor sheaths in the hand. (1)

4. What sites other than the hand can be affected by Dupuytren's disease?(2)

5. Dupuytren's contractures when severe cause exquisite pain. (1)

6. Where are Garrod's pads?(1)

7. In Volkmann's ischaemic contracture the fingers are held in permanent flexion or clawing. (1)

8. Mallet finger is a result of extensor tendon rupture at the distal phalanx. (1)

9. Extensor pollicis longus may rupture spontaneously at the wrist in rheumatoid arthritis. (1)

10. Boutonnière deformity involves flexion at the distal interphalangeal joint and extension at the proximal interphalangeal joint. (1)

11. Swan-neck deformity is most commonly seen in rheumatoid arthritis. (1)

12. Thickening of the fibrous tendon sheath causes stenosing tenovaginitis. (1)

Answers opposite

The Hand

1. False: it is the ability to identify and name objects by touch alone.

2. True

3. False: it is thickening of the palmar aponeurosis and palmar fascia.

4. The feet – thickening of the plantar fascia. There is also an association with Peyronie's disease (fibrosis of the corpus cavernosum of the penis).

5. False: pain is very rarely a feature.

6. On the knuckles of those affected by Dupuytren's disease.

7. False: flexion of the wrist will allow straightening of the fingers. The disorder is due to a shortening of the muscle–tendon unit.

8. True

9. True: repair is effected by transferring the extensor indicis tendon from the index finger to the thumb.

10. False: the deformity described is known as a 'swan-neck'. Boutonnière deformity is due to rupture of the central slip of the extensor tendon to produce flexion at the proximal inter-phalangeal joint and extension at the distal interphalangeal joint.

11. True

12. True: thickening follows local trauma or unaccustomed activity.

13. In rheumatoid arthritis, the fingers develop ulnar subluxation at the metacarpophalangeal joints. (1)

14. Periarticular erosions seen on X-ray are characteristic of late rheumatoid disease in the hand. (1)

15. Heberden's nodes are a poor prognostic sign in rheumatoid arthritis. (1)

16. A whitlow is pulp space infection of the finger. (1)

17. Tendon sheath infections may result in a stiff useless finger. (1)

18. Tendon sheath infection in the middle and ring fingers may track up into the wrist. (1)

19. The position in which the hand should be splinted is 90° flexion of proximal interphalangeal joints with metacarpophalangeal and distal interphalangeal joints extended. (1)

20. The position of splintage referred to in the answer to Question 19 allows relaxation of the capsular ligaments to prevent stretching. (1)

21. Extensor tendon injuries are more demanding to repair than flexor injuries. (1)

Total score	22
Target score	
Postgraduate	20
Undergraduate	17

Answers opposite

13. True: this is 'ulnar drift'.

14. True: due to the erosive effect of inflamed synovium on the underlying osteoporotic bone.

15. False: they are associated with osteoarthritis.

16. True

17. True: unless drainage of pus is affected at an early stage and mobility of the finger is maintained.

18. False: the thumb and little finger are the only digits with tendon sheaths extending into the wrist.

19. False: the metacarpophalangeal joints should be flexed to 90°, and the proximal and distal interphalangeal joints extended.

20. False: the position maintains the ligaments taut, so if they do become adherent, a good range of movement may be recovered.

21. False: deep and superficial flexor tendons are in close proximity, and run in a complex system of sheaths and pulleys which renders the repair more difficult.

The Neck

1. Traction on the arm in a patient with a tight thoracic outlet weakens the radial pulse. (1)

2. A single anteroposterior and lateral X-ray of the neck are sufficient to show the cervical vertebrae. (1)

3. Instability of the cervical spine can be demonstrated by X-rays. (1)

4. Congenital torticollis arises due to a deformity in the sterno-mastoid muscle. (1)

5. Prolapse of a cervical disc most commonly occurs at the level of C2/3. (1)

6. Oblique views of the neck are used to show the intervertebral foramina. (1)

7. Inflamed cervical lymph nodes may cause secondary torticollis. (1)

8. Cervical disc pathology commonly causes occipital headache. (1)

9. Neuralgic amyotrophy usually causes pain in the neck. (1)

10. Cervical disc prolapse needs urgent surgical removal. (1)

11. Cervical spondylosis is the most common of all cervical spine disorders. (1)

Answers opposite

The Neck

1. True: if the thoracic outlet is abnormally tight then traction may cause the pulse to weaken or disappear.

2. False: an anteroposterior projection through the open mouth is needed to show the first two vertebrae. Considerable traction may be needed on the arms in the lateral view to show the lower cervical vertebrae.

3. True: this requires lateral films in flexion and extension.

4. True: the sternomastoid on one side is fibrous and fails to elongate as the neck grows, thus twisting the chin to the opposite side.

5. False: the most common site of disc prolapse is above or below the 6th cervical vertebra and may thus affect the nerve roots of C6 or C7.

6. True

7. True

8. True

9. False: the pain is usually felt around the shoulder but may radiate to the neck and give a clinical picture similar to cervical disc disease or spondylosis.

10. False: conservative treatment using a collar and traction may allow symptoms to settle. When the symptoms remain severe then the disc can be removed surgically via an anterior approach and the disc space grafted.

11. True

12. X-ray changes of cervical spondylosis usually signify severe symptoms. (1)

13. Osteophytes in cervical spondylosis may cause pressure on the nerve roots as they exit from the intervertebral foramina. (1)

14. Disc space height is usually maintained in cervical spondylosis. (1)

15. Physiotherapy gives symptomatic relief in the majority of cases of cervical spondylosis. (1)

16. Involvement of the cervical spine is a rare complication of rheumatoid arthritis. (1)

17. In rheumatoid arthritis of the neck atlantoaxial instability may occur due to synovitis. (1)

18. Neurological complications are common with rheumatoid cervical spine instability. (1)

19. The pain of neuralgic amyotrophy usually settles within a few days. (1)

20. Neuralgic amyotrophy is caused by a viral infection of the nerve roots. (1)

Total score   20
Target score
    Postgraduate   18
    Undergraduate   15

Answers opposite

12. False: the X-ray changes of cervical spondylosis are a relatively common incidental finding and there are often no symptoms.

13. True: these are best seen in oblique X-rays which show the intervertebral foramina.

14. False: the involved area, usually C5–6, shows narrowing of the disc spaces in the lateral film and small bony spurs on the anterior corners of the vertebrae.

15. True

16. False: the cervical spine is seriously affected in 30% of patients with rheumatoid arthritis.

17. True: there is synovitis of the lateral atlantoaxial joints and around the odontoid which causes erosion of the transverse ligaments and allows forward subluxation of C1 (atlas) on C2 (axis). This may be asymptomatic but should be suspected in all patients with rheumatoid arthritis undergoing surgery. Prior to general anaesthesia flexion and extension views of the neck should be taken to assess stability.

18. False: neurological complications are surprisingly uncommon and most cases can be managed conservatively with a collar. Instability that is severe or progressive or causing neurological deficit can be stabilized surgically by posterior fusion.

19. True: the severe pain settles within a few days but full recovery of neurological function may take months or years.

20. True: this is believed to be the aetiology.

The Back

1. Abnormal patches of hair on the back indicate an increased likelihood of disc prolapse. (1)

2. Rotation of the spine occurs mainly at the thoracic vertebra. (1)

3. In disc prolapse the straight leg raise on the unaffected side may cause pain in the opposite leg. (1)

4. Mobile scoliosis may be caused by vertebral abnormality. (1)

5. The thoracic curve in adolescent idiopathic scoliosis is convex to the right in the majority of cases. (1)

6. Neurofibromatosis may be associated with spinal deformity. (1)

7. Infantile scoliosis is the most common type of scoliosis. (1)

8. In scoliosis lumbar curves produce less cosmetic deformity than thoracic curves. (1)

9. Operative treatment is preferred for curves over 30°. (1)

10. Scheuermann's disease affects mainly adolescent boys. (1)

11. Scheuermann's disease produces wedging of the vertebral bodies anteriorly. (1)

12. The spine is the third most common site for bony tuberculosis. (1)

13. The Mantoux test is usually negative in spinal tuberculosis. (1)

14. Spinal tuberculosis may cause spinal cord damage. (1)

Answers opposite

The Back

1. False: abnormal hairy patches indicate the possibility of a vertebral arch malformation such as spina bifida.

2. True: flexion occurs mainly at the cervical and lumbar regions.

3. True: this is crossed sciatic tension and indicates severe root irritation.

4. False: in mobile scoliosis there is no structural abnormality and the curve is reversible.

5. True: this is the case in 90% of patients.

6. True: although the cause is unknown.

7. False: the commonest type is adolescent idiopathic scoliosis.

8. True: thoracic deformities are associated with a rib prominence and unequal shoulders. Lumbar curves often pass unnoticed.

9. False: these may be successfully treated in braces. Operative treatment is usually reserved for those over 45°.

10. False: it is twice as common in girls.

11. True: due to a disorder in the vertebral growth plate.

12. False: it is the most common.

13. False

14. True: collapse of the vertebral bodies may damage the cord in the spinal canal.

15. Abscess formation in spinal tuberculosis must be treated with continuous antituberculous chemotherapy for 6 months. (1)

16. L4/5 and L5/S1 are the most common sites for disc prolapse. (1)

17. If bladder control is lost following a lumbar disc protrusion, this commonly resolves after 3 weeks' bed rest. (1)

18. Reduced ankle jerk indicates S1 root impingement. (1)

19. Most cases of disc prolapse resolve with bed rest. (1)

20. Posterior facet joint osteoarthritis follows recurrent disc prolapse. (1)

21. Spinal stenosis may produce symptoms in one leg only. (1)

22. Symptoms of spinal stenosis are relieved by squatting. (1).

23. Spondylolisthesis describes a backwards shift of one vertebra on the one below. (1)

24. L3/L4 level is the most common area for spondylolisthesis. (1)

Total 24
Target score
    Postgraduate 21
    Undergraduate 18

Answers opposite

15. False: the presence of an abscess is an indication for surgical drainage.

16. True

17. False: loss of bladder control is a surgical emergency requiring immediate decompression of the sacral roots.

18. True

19. True: approximately 90% of patients recover.

20. True: due to loss of disc height, abnormal forces act upon the facet joint, producing osteoarthritic change.

21. True: this is root canal stenosis.

22. True: flexing the spine reduces cord compression in the canal.

23. False: it is a forwards shift.

24. False: spondylolisthesis occurs most commonly at the L5/S1 level.

The Hip

1. A painful knee may be the only symptom of hip pathology. (1)

2. Pain from the hip is often felt behind the joint. (1)

3. A Trendelenburg test is positive if the unsupported side of the pelvis rises. (1)

4. Apparent shortening occurs in fixed abduction of the hip. (1)

5. Fixed flexion is tested by fully flexing the contralateral hip. (1)

6. Hip rotation can be assessed with the hip flexed or extended. (1)

7. Both legs must be in a similar position with respect to the pelvis for true leg lengths to be assessed. (1)

8. Shortening of the femur above the greater trochanter cannot be determined clinically. (1)

9. Apparent length is measured from the anterior superior iliac spine to the medial malleolus. (1)

10. Hip extension is normally less than 10°. (1).

11. 'Telescoping' of the hip is a normal finding. (1)

12. Shenton's line connects the greater and lesser trochanters. (1)

13. Congenital dislocation of the hip occurs in 2% of newborn babies. (1)

Answers opposite

The Hip

1. True: this is well known, but often forgotten and a normal knee is subjected to fruitless investigation.

2. False: pain felt behind the hip usually derives from the lumbar spine. Pain from the hip is felt in the groin.

3. False: in a positive Trendelenburg test the unsupported side drops due to abductor weakness, bony instability or pain.

4. False: fixed abduction makes the leg appear long.

5. True: this is the basis of Thomas's test for fixed flexion. Flexion of the contralateral hip neutralizes any pelvic tilt and reveals any fixed hip flexion this may have concealed.

6. True

7. True

8. False: it can be estimated by feeling the height of the greater trochanters with respect to the anterior superior iliac spines.

9. False: this is the way to measure true length.

10. True

11. False: it denotes marked instability.

12. False: it is a line which continues from the inferior border of the neck of the femur to the inferior border of the superior pubic ramus. Any interruption in the curve of this line suggests an abnormality of the hip.

13. False: the incidence is about 2 in 1000 (0.2%).

14. Congenital dislocation of the hip is bilateral in approximately one third of cases. (1)

15. Congenital dislocation is more common in American Indians. (1)

16. The femoral neck is usually retroverted in congenital dislocation of the hip. (1)

17. In congenital dislocation of the hip there is no abnormality of the acetabulum. (1)

18. Unilateral dislocation of the hip in infants is easier to diagnose than bilateral hip dislocation. (1)

19. X-rays in congenital dislocation of the hip show the femoral head epiphysis to be displaced upwards and outwards. (1)

20. Ortolani's sign is a clunk denoting reduction of the dislocated hip. (1)

21. Treatment of congenital dislocation of the hip or unstable hips in the newborn consists of maintaining the hip in the abducted position. (1)

22. Bilateral congenital dislocation of the hip, when discovered after the age of 6, is often not treated. (1)

23. Acquired dislocation of hip may occur in children with unbalanced muscle paralysis if the hip abductors are weaker than the adductors. (1)

24. The 'television position' is associated with femoral neck anteversion. (1)

Answers opposite

14. True: it is also more common in females and on the left side.

15. True: because they swaddle their babies with hips extended.

16. False: it is often anteverted.

17. False: it is usually shallow.

18. True: this is because in bilateral congenital dislocation of the hip there is no asymmetry and the waddling gait may be mistaken for toddling.

19. True: but X-rays may be of little value in the newborn because the head is entirely cartilaginous and not visible radiographically. Ultrasound scanning shows promise as a newer imaging technique.

20. True: Barlow's sign is the reverse. Both are useful clinical tests for congenital dislocation of the hip.

21. True: by using double nappies, a von Rosen splint or a Pavlik harness.

22. True

23. True: this may occur in conditions such as cerebral palsy.

24. True: in this position the child sits on the floor with both knees bent and both hips in full internal rotation.

25. Protrusio acetabuli normally occurs at birth. (1)

26. The essential lesion in Perthes' disease is an avascular necrosis of the femoral head. (1)

27. The earliest stages of Perthes' disease can be assessed using X-rays. (1)

28. Perthes' disease is more common in girls. (1)

29. Perthes' disease usually presents with a limp or hip pain. (1)

30. Prognosis in Perthes' disease is independent of the amount of femoral head involved. (1)

31. Children with Perthes' disease who have favourable prognostic signs do not need active treatment. (1)

32. Children with unfavourable prognostic signs in Perthes' disease need surgery. (1)

33. Slipped upper femoral epiphysis usually occurs suddenly following trauma. (1)

34. Slipped upper femoral epiphysis tends to occur in children who are short or thin with precocious puberty. (1)

35. Slipped upper femoral epiphysis is more common in girls than in boys. (1)

36. Slipped upper femoral epiphysis commonly presents with pain in the knee. (1)

Answers opposite

25. False: it is usually acquired. Women are more commonly affected than men and it is associated with diseases that cause softening of the bone such as osteomalacia, Paget's and long-standing rheumatoid arthritis.

26. True

27. False: X-rays may be normal in the early stages but bone scans and magnetic resonance imaging can demonstrate ischaemic areas of the femoral head.

28. False: it is four times more common in boys.

29. True

30. False: Catterall has devised a prognostic grading system of I–IV depending on the extent of femoral head involvement.

31. True: they should, however, be followed up. The term 'supervised neglect' is an apt description!

32. False: treatment is by containment of the femoral head in the acetabulum to retain its normal shape. This may be achieved by long term abduction splintage or by osteotomy of the femur or pelvis.

33. False: 70% of cases are chronic slips occurring gradually.

34. False: the opposite, it often occurs in children who are tall, fat and with delayed development.

35. False

36. True

37. Examination of a patient with slipped upper femoral epiphysis reveals the leg to be short and externally rotated. (1)

38. Trethowan's line is drawn along the inferior aspect of the neck of the femur. (1)

39. Give two complications of slipped upper femoral epiphysis. (2)

40. Slipped upper femoral epiphysis is best treated by manipulation under anaesthetic. (1)

41. Pyogenic arthritis of the hip is usually seen in children under the age of 2. (1)

42. In pyogenic arthritis of the hip the commonest organism is *Staphylococcus aureus*. (1)

43. In the early stages of pyogenic arthritis of the hip X-rays are more helpful than ultrasound. (1)

44. A patient with pyogenic arthritis should have open arthrotomy and lavage performed as soon as possible. (1)

45. Healed tuberculosis of the hip often results in fibrous ankylosis. (1)

46. Osteophyte formation commonly occurs in rheumatoid arthritis of the hip. (1)

47. Rheumatoid arthritis of the hip may show rapid erosion of the femoral head. (1)

Answers opposite

37. True

38. False: it is drawn along the superior aspect of the neck in an anteroposterior X-ray and in normal children intersects the femoral epiphysis. In slipped upper femoral epiphysis the line passes above the epiphysis.

39. Any of:
Avascular necrosis of the femoral head
Coxa vara
Chondrolysis
Secondary osteoarthritis
Slipping of the other side

40. False: this carries a high risk of causing avascular necrosis and is not recommended. If the slip is minor it can be pinned *in situ*. Greater slips may need more complex surgery to realign the head and neck.

41. True: it is a very serious condition as the cartilaginous femoral head can be rapidly destroyed by the proteolytic enzymes of bacteria and pus.

42. True

43. False: X-rays are usually unchanged but ultrasound scanning may show an effusion.

44. True

45. True

46. False

47. True

48. List four predisposing causes of secondary osteoarthritis of the hip. (4)

49. Primary osteoarthritis is so called because no underlying cause has been discovered. (1)

50. In osteoarthritis of the hip pain is characteristically worse on initiating movement and may then ease off. (1)

51. Stiffness is seldom a problem in osteoarthritis of the hip. (1)

52. In osteoarthritis of the hip the leg is usually shortened and internally rotated. (1)

53. List four X-ray features of osteoarthritis. (4)

54. Early osteoarthritis is best treated with total hip replacement before deformity develops. (1)

55. Patients with X-ray evidence of severe osteoarthritis of the hip are best treated with total hip replacement. (1)

56. Osteotomy of the proximal femur is often of benefit in young patients with osteoarthritis. (1)

57. Total hip replacement is a treatment better suited to patients under 55. (1)

Total		64
Target score		
Postgraduate		59
Undergraduate		52

Answers opposite

48. Any four from:
     Congenital dislocation of the hip
     Perthes' disease
     Coxa vara
     Acetabular deformities
     Injury
     Rheumatoid arthritis
     Avascular necrosis
     Paget's disease
     Infective arthritis

49. True

50. True

51. False: lack of hip flexion often means the patient cannot reach to put on socks or cut his or her toe nails.

52. False: it is usually shortened, externally rotated and adducted.

53. Decreased joint space
Subarticular sclerosis
Cyst formation
Osteophytes

54. False: conservative methods should be employed primarily.

55. False: treatment must be based on the patient and symptoms and not the X-rays.

56. True: realignment of the femoral head allows redistribution of stress to a less damaged part of the joint. Venous hypertension is thought to play a part in the pain of osteoarthritis and osteotomy also helps to relieve this.

57. False: total hip replacement has a limited life span and the more active life style of younger patients means the prosthesis wears out or is loosened more quickly.

The Knee

1. What are the important questions to ask about the knee when taking a history?(6)

2. What should you *look* at when examining a knee?(3)

3. What tests for fluid in the knee do you know?(3)

4. What is the medical term for 'bow legs'?(1)

5. Give three causes of 'bow legs'. (3)

6. Which meniscus is most commonly injured and why?(2)

Answers opposite

The Knee

1. Ask about:
   injury, if any
   pain
   stiffness
   swelling
   locking
   giving way

2. You should look at:

   the skin   – colour
                  – scars
                  – sinuses

   the shape   – muscle wasting
                    – swelling
                    – lumps
                    – patella shape and position

   the position   – valgus/varus (check this standing)
                      – flexed/hyperextended

3. Cross fluctuation   – for a large effusion

   Patellar tap   – for a moderate effusion

   The bulge test (also known as the wipe test)
           – for a small effusion.

4. Genu varum.

5. Any three from
   Physiological   – in babies
   Epiphyseal disorders e.g. Blount's disease
   Metaphyseal disorders e.g. dyschondroplasia
   Post-traumatic   – following fractures or epiphyseal plate
                            injuries
   Metabolic disorders, e.g. rickets, arthritis, Paget's disease.

6. The medial because it is more tightly attached to the tibial plateau than the lateral and therefore less mobile.

7. Which two tests are useful in the diagnosis of a torn meniscus?(2)

8. Tears of the menisci seldom heal. (1)

9. What is the most common mode of injury to produce a meniscal tear?(1)

10. Give three clinical features associated with meniscal injury of the knee. (3)

11. The effusion associated with meniscal injury arises immediately after injury. (1)

12. Osgood–Schlatter's disease is a traction effect on the tibial apophysis. There is no radiographic changes. (1)

13. Osteochondritis dissecans affects patients 15–20 years old. (1)

14. In osteochondritis dissecans, a small osteochondral fragment usually separates from the lateral femoral condyle. (1)

15. Give three predisposing causes for recurrent dislocation of the patella. (3)

16. A teenage girl complaining of anterior knee pain worsened by climbing stairs and exercise may be suffering from what condition?(1)

17. Synovitis precedes articular damage in rheumatoid disease of the knee. (1)

Answers opposite

7. McMurray's test.
   Apley's grinding test – this test will also differentiate between meniscal and ligament damage.

8. True: the vast majority don't heal and require surgery. However, peripheral tears in the more vascular areas of the meniscus may heal.

9. Characteristically a twisting force on a flexed knee. Commonly occurs in football.

10. Three of: pain, effusion, locking, fixed flexion deformity.

11. False: it often arises some hours later, or the following day.

12. False: it is a traction effect, but radiographs may show fragmentation of the tibial apophysis. Spontaneous recovery is normal.

13. True

14. False: probably as a result of trauma there is an osteochondral fracture, but it is most commonly from the *medial condyle*.

15. Any three from: generalized ligamentous laxity, anatomical deformities of the patella, e.g. patella alta, valgus deformity of the knee, hypoplasia of the lateral femoral condyle.

16. Chondromalacia patellae. The condition usually resolves spontaneously after 2 or 3 years, and is due to softening of the retropatella cartilage.

17. True

18. Give four predisposing factors in osteoarthritis of the knee. (4)

19. What pathognomonic sign do you look for in recurrent dislocation of the patella?(1)

20. Give three modes of conservative management of the osteoarthritic knee. (3)

21. Prepatellar bursitis is a common affliction of carpet layers and plumbers. (1)

22. What two operative procedures may be performed for isolated medial compartment osteoarthritis of the knee?(2)

Total score	45
Target score	
Postgraduate	42
Undergraduate	38

Answers opposite

18. Trauma – fractures round the knee and meniscal injuries
    Abnormal stresses e.g. joint deformity or obesity
    Subchondral bony abnormalities e.g. osteonecrosis
    Previous inflammatory or infective arthritis.

19. The apprehension sign. Patients become apprehensive when the patella is pushed laterally.

20. Analgesics
    Non-steroidal anti-inflammatory drugs
    Physiotherapy
    Walking aids if required.

21. True: inflammation and infection of the prepatellar bursa occur due to the constant friction between the skin and the patella. This condition is seen most often in those whose occupation involves prolonged work on the knees.

22. Upper tibial osteotomy of the tibia to 'offload' the medial compartment.
    Medial compartment knee replacement.

The Ankle and Foot

1. Metatarsalgia is often associated with muscle fatigue. (1)

2. Palpation of the foot is best performed with the patient standing. (1)

3. Eversion and inversion of the foot take place at the midtarsal joint. (1)

4. What is the Latin name for congenital club foot?(1)

5. Congenital club foot is more common in girls. (1)

6. Congenital club foot is usually bilateral. (1)

7. Congenital club foot is associated with arthrogryphosis. (1)

8. Club foot usually resolves with growth. (1)

9. In congenital club foot the talus points upwards. (1)

10. In congenital club foot the heel and calf are often reduced in size. (1)

11. Congenital club foot is treated within 2 or 3 days of birth by strapping specifically to correct the equinus deformity. (1)

12. Surgery should not be performed in cases of congenital club foot that are resistant to treatment by stretching and splinting. (1)

13. In children over the age of 10 correction of club foot usually requires bony as well as soft tissue procedures. (1)

Answers opposite

The Ankle and Foot

1. True

2. False: it is best performed when the patient is sitting.

3. False: they mainly occur at the subtalar joint.

4. Talipes equinovarus.

5. False: it is twice as common in boys.

6. False: it is bilateral in one third of cases.

7. True: it is also associated with myelomeningocele.

8. False: it often deteriorates as secondary growth changes occur in the bones.

9. False: it points downwards.

10. True

11. False: the forefoot adduction should be corrected first, then the supination and only last the equinus. Over-zealous attempts to correct equinus may break the foot in the midtarsal region causing a 'rocker bottom' deformity.

12. False: this is an indication for surgery which essentially comprises release of the tight posterior medial structures followed by splintage.

13. True

14. Flat foot is abnormal in children of 1–2 years. (1)

15. Most flat feet do not require surgical treatment. (1)

16. Pes cavus is associated with claw toes. (1)

17. In pes cavus pain is often felt in the high instep. (1)

18. Most cases of pes cavus require surgical correction. (1)

19. Hallux valgus is associated with valgus of the first metatarsal. (1)

20. Only the big toe is deformed in hallux valgus. (1)

21. In hallux valgus the big toe is often rotated medially. (1)

22. Hallux valgus is most common in teenage girls. (1)

23. Hallux valgus predisposes to secondary osteoarthritis of the first metatarsophalangeal joint. (1)

24. In hallux valgus X-rays of the foot should be taken with the patient sitting. (1)

25. Surgical treatment of hallux valgus in young people is aimed at correcting the varus deformity of the first metatarsal. (1)

26. Hallux rigidus is a condition involving osteoarthritis of the interphalangeal joint of the big toe. (1)

27. Hallux rigidus may be treated by a stiff rocker-soled shoe. (1)

Answers opposite

14. False: most children appear to be flat-footed when they start walking.

15. True

16. True: this may be due to weak or unbalanced intrinsic muscles.

17. False: pain is more commonly felt under the metatarsal heads or over the toes where shoe pressure is most marked.

18. False: most need no treatment.

19. False: it is associated with a varus deformity of the first metatarsal, the so-called metatarsus primus varus.

20. False: the big toe deviates towards the second toe which may become secondarily deformed. There may also be hammer-toe deformities of the other digits.

21. True

22. False: it is most common in women over 50.

23. True

24. False: the patient should be standing in order to show the deformity on weight bearing.

25. True

26. False: it is the metatarsophalangeal joint that is affected.

27. True: this allows the foot to roll without any dorsiflexion at the metatarsophalangeal joint.

28. Most cases of claw toes are due to an underlying neurological abnormality. (1)

29. Fixed claw toes can be treated by transferring the long flexors to the extensors. (1)

30. The foot and ankle are seldom affected by rheumatoid arthritis. (1)

31. Rupture of the tibialis posterior can lead to valgus deformity of the ankle. (1)

32. Swelling of the metatarsophalangeal joints, flattened arches, claw toes and hallux valgus are characteristic of osteoarthritis of the forefoot. (1)

33. Simmond's test demonstrates an intact Achilles tendon if the ankle dorsiflexes when the calf is squeezed. (1)

34. Rupture of the tendo Achilles occurs most commonly in the young. (1)

35. Treatment of tendo Achilles rupture can be either conservative or surgical. (1)

36. Sever's disease describes painful spurs under the heel. (1)

37. Kohler's disease describes osteochondritis of the talus. (1)

38. Freiberg's disease describes osteochondritis of the head of the second metatarsal. (1)

39. Stress fractures commonly occur in the metatarsals. (1)

Answers opposite

28. False: this is true in a few cases, but in the majority no cause is found.

29. False: this procedure may work when the joints can be passively corrected, but once they become stiff tendon transfer must be combined with interphalangeal arthrodesis.

30. False

31. True: this may occur in the late stages of rheumatoid arthritis.

32. False: these are characteristic of rheumatoid arthritis.

33. False: the ankle plantar flexes if the tendon is intact. If it is ruptured the foot and ankle remain still.

34. False: it is most common in the over 40s when the tendon is more degenerate.

35. True: a cast with the ankle in equinus is needed in both cases to protect the healing tendon for at least 8 weeks.

36. False: Sever's disease describes a traction apophysitis of the insertion of the tendo Achilles into the calcaneus. It usually occurs in boys of about 10.

37. False: it is osteochondritis of the navicular.

38. True

39. True

40. Morton's metatarsalgia is a painful condition of the forefoot of unknown aetiology. (1)

41. Ingrowing toenail may be treated by wedge resection. (1)

42. Onychogryphosis is usually caused by subungual exostosis. (1)

Total score	42
Target score	
Postgraduate	39
Undergraduate	33

Answers opposite

40. False: it is indeed a painful condition of the forefoot caused by a sensitive neuroma of the digital nerve in the 3rd or 4th clefts.

41. True: this is one of many operations to alleviate this condition.

42. False

Fracture Pathology and Diagnosis

1. A compound fracture consists of many fragments. (1)

2. In order to fracture, the bone must be subject to a force greater than its tensile strength. (1)

3. Pathological fractures are produced by a minimal force. (1)

4. Spiral fractures are produced by a twisting force. (1)

5. Greenstick fractures are characteristically seen in haemophiliacs. (1)

6. Muscle spasm may cause angulation or rotation of a fracture. (1)

7. Osteoclasts are cells which produce bone. (1)

8. A healed fracture will remodel its shape for many months following the injury. (1)

9. Cortical bone heals faster than cancellous bone. (1)

10. Non-union of a fracture may be produced by soft tissue separating the bone ends. (1)

11. In fractures of the forearm joints above and below the injury should be included in the X-ray. (1)

12. Callus usually appears earlier in lower limb fractures.

Total	12
Target score	
Postgraduate	11
Undergraduate	9

Answers opposite

Fracture Pathology and Diagnosis

1. False: 'compound' implies the skin over the fracture is breached and the fracture is open.

2. False: small forces, repeated often, will lead to stress fractures, e.g. fibula or tibia.

3. True: due to a pathological process in the bone, it is greatly weakened.

4. True

5. False: they occur in children.

6. True

7. False: they cause bone reabsorption.

8. True

9. False

10. True

11. True

12. False: callus appears at the same time, irrespective of the site of the fracture.

Principles of Fracture Treatment

1. The first priority in first aid to the severely injured is to stop any bleeding using local compression. (1)

2. Treatment of fractures should be undertaken before the patient is resuscitated. (1)

3. Fracture healing is impaired by muscle activity and weight bearing. (1)

4. In reducing a long bone fracture alignment of the fragments is more important than apposition. (1)

5. Fractures involving an articular surface need not be accurately reduced. (1)

6. Open reduction should be used if soft tissue interposition between fragments prevents closed reduction. (1)

7. Fractures are splinted to ensure union. (1)

8. Traction can be discontinued in favour of functional bracing as soon as the fracture shows signs of uniting. (1)

9. Skin traction can be used to produce a pull of up to 20 kg. (1)

10. Joint stiffness is seldom a problem after immobilization in a plaster cast. (1)

11. Plasters should not be split after manipulation of closed fractures or displacement of the fragments may occur. (1)

12. Pressure sores under plaster casts are usually caused because weight bearing is started too early. (1)

Answers opposite

Principles of Fracture Treatment

1. False: it is to make sure the airway is clear.

2. False

3. False: it is promoted by both of these.

4. True

5. False: accurate reduction should be attempted as any irregularity in the articular surface will predispose to degenerative arthritis.

6. True

7. False: fractures are splinted to alleviate pain and to ensure that union occurs in a position of good function.

8. True

9. False: the accepted limit is around 5 kg. Forces greater than this should use skeletal traction.

10. False: it is a common problem and one of the main drawbacks with this method of treatment.

11. False: splitting is commonly performed to allow swelling of the underlying tissues and to avoid the cast acting as a tourniquet.

12. False: it is usually localized pressure from the cast that causes pressure sores. These should be avoided by adequate padding.

13. Functional braces for femoral fractures are best applied within the first few days of the injury. (1)

14. Weight bearing is safe once a fracture has been internally fixed. (1)

15. Prophylactic antibiotics should be given before internal fixation. (1)

16. The commonest cause of osteomyelitis today is surgery. (1)

The following questions 17–21 are indications for internal fixation

17. Fractures in athletes. (1)

18. Fractures that are inherently unstable. (1)

19. Pathological fractures. (1)

20. Fractures of the dominant forearm. (1)

21. Multiple limb injuries. (1)

22. Non-union of the forearm is more likely to occur if both radius and ulna are broken. (1)

23. Following internal fixation, the metalwork is best left *in situ* for at least a year. (1)

24. External fixation should be avoided where there is severe soft tissue damage. (1)

Answers opposite

13. False: they should not be applied until union has started to occur, i.e. after 4–6 weeks of traction or conventional cast.

14. False: there are some types of fractures and fixation methods that allow immediate weight bearing, e.g. transverse femoral and tibial fractures fixed with intramedullary nails, however in general weight bearing should not be allowed until the bone itself has united.

15. True: most surgeons would agree with this.

16. True

17. False

18. True

19. True

20. False

21. True

22. False: it is more likely if only one bone is fractured as the intact bone may hold the fractured end apart.

23. True

24. False: this is in fact one of its prime indications as the damaged tissue can be inspected.

25. Oedema following fractures of the hand should be treated by elevation and exercise of the fingers. (1)

26. Passive movement of joints following internal fixation should be avoided. (1)

27. Open fractures should be treated by early surgery to clean the wound. (1)

28. Patients with compound fractures should be given antibiotics. (1)

29. Devitalized tissue in the wounds of open fractures should be carefully observed over the following 5 days. (1)

30. Skin edges of wounds in contaminated fractures should be carefully trimmed by excising a thin margin. (1)

31. Contaminated wounds should, in general, be debrided and sutured as soon as possible. (1)

32. Delayed primary closure of contaminated wounds should be carried out at 24 hours. (1)

33. Salter Harris type 2 epiphyseal injuries often result in abnormal growth patterns. (1)

Total score   33
Total target
    Postgraduate   31
    Undergraduate   28

Answers opposite

25. True

26. False: this has been taught in the past but is not true. Forced movements should be avoided especially at the elbow, but gentle passive assistance, e.g. on continuous passive motion machines, can be helpful in regaining function after injuries.

27. True: this should take place within 6 hours.

28. True: tetanus prophylaxis should also be considered.

29. False: this is a source of infection and should be excised at early operation.

30. True

31. False: delayed primary closure of these wounds should be performed, provided they remain clean.

32. False: delayed primary suture should not be carried out until at least 5 days from injury.

33. False: types 1 and 2 seldom result in serious growth problems. Types 3–5, however, are likely to result in deformities due to premature growth arrest.

Complications of Fractures

1. Neurogenic shock occurs when bleeding occurs into the central nervous system. (1)

2. Patients in oligaemic shock often complain of thirst. (1)

3. Renal failure is a recognized complication of injuries in which a limb is crushed for several hours. (1)

4. In the crush syndrome collagen is released from muscle which causes blockage of the renal tubules. (1)

5. Homan's sign is pain on dorsiflexing the ankle and is positive in thrombosis of the femoral veins. (1)

6. Pelvic and femoral venous thrombosis has a higher tendency to produce pulmonary embolism than thrombosis of the calf veins. (1)

7. The tetanus organism invades the anterior horn cells to produce paralysis. (1)

8. Human antitoxin to tetanus, if administered rapidly, reverses the paralytic effects. (1)

9. *Clostridium welchii* produces gas gangrene. (1)

10. Gas formation within infected tissues is a pathognomonic sign of gas gangrene. (1)

11. In gas gangrene, antitoxin should be administered immediately. (1)

12. Fat embolism syndrome occurs most commonly after a long bone fracture. (1)

Answers opposite

Complications of Fractures

1. False: in neurogenic shock there is no loss of blood volume but its distribution is faulty, with excess blood volume in the non-essential circulation.

2. True

3. True: this is the crush syndrome.

4. False

5. False: Homan's sign is positive if the thrombosis is situated in the calf veins.

6. True: anticoagulants are strongly indicated.

7. False: the tetanus organism remains in the wound. The effects on the anterior horn cells are produced by an exotoxin.

8. False: once the paralysis has occurred, antitoxin does not reverse the process.

9. True

10. False: other forms of anaerobic cellulitis may also cause gas formation wihtin tissues.

11. False: there is no antitoxin.

12. True: although fat embolism may follow a fracture of any bone.

13. Fat embolism syndrome causes a decrease in blood Po_2 even if there is no associated chest injury. (1)

14. Infection at a fracture site always prevents union. (1)

15. A painless pseudoarthrosis may develop at the site of non-union. (1)

16. A malunion causing shortening of the lower limb by 1 cm requires realignment. (1)

17. Epiphyseal injuries in children are associated with deformities in later life. (1)

18. Avascular necrosis may follow fracture of the neck of the talus. (1)

19. Fractured limbs associated with a vascular injury should be rested until swelling decreases and the pulses return. (1)

20. Name an investigation useful in diagnosing vascular injury. (1)

21. Compartment syndrome may be diagnosed when the pulses distal to the compression are absent. (1)

22. Myositis ossificans occurs after infection of muscle. (1)

Answers opposite

13. True: although the exact pathogenesis is unclear.

14. False: not always. Many fractures will heal in the presence of infection, although the healing may be delayed.

15. True: this is produced by interposition of fibrous tissue at the fracture site.

16. False: shortening of more than 2.5 cm requires treatment; 1 cm is not significant.

17. True: angulation at the growth plate causes limbs to develop abnormally.

18. True: other recognized sites for avascular necrosis are the head of the femur and the proximal part of the scaphoid.

19. False: vascular injury following a fracture is a surgical emergency. It should be treated immediately.

20. One of: angiography or Doppler ultrasound.

21. False: the best diagnostic test is in increase in pain when the toes or fingers are hyperextended. The presence of a pulse does not exclude the diagnosis.

22. False: it usually occurs after muscle trauma, characteristically around the elbow.

23. Joint stiffness may follow immobilization of the fractured limb, even though the joint is not involved in the fracture. (1)

24. Osteoarthritis is a recognized complication of a fracture involving the articular surface. (1)

25. Sudeck's atrophy (reflex sympathetic dystrophy) most commonly affects the foot or hand. (1)

26. The more severe injuries are most likely to get Sudeck's atrophy. (1)

Total	26
Target score	
Postgraduate	23
Undergraduate	20

Answers opposite

23. True

24. True

25. True: although it may affect any injured joint.

26. False: often the injury is relatively minor.

Stress Fractures and Pathological Fractures

1. A stress fracture is one caused by a single stress of sufficient strength to break the bone. (1)

2. The 'march fracture' is a stress fracture of the fibula. (1)

3. Stress fracture of the pars interarticularis is found in precocious gymnasts. (1)

4. Stress fractures are easily diagnosed on X-rays. (1)

5. Stress fractures should be treated with internal fixation. (1)

6. Pathological fractures only occur in abnormal or diseased bone. (1)

7. Biopsy may be necessary for diagnosis in pathological fractures.

8. Treatment of pathological fractures commonly involves internal fixation. (1)

9. The underlying bone disorder can be ignored in the treatment of pathological fractures. (1)

10. If isolated metastatic deposits from a known primary tumour are found in long bones, these should be treated with prophylactic internal fixation. (1)

Total score	10	
Target score		
Postgraduate	9	
Undergraduate	8	

Answers opposite

Stress Fractures and Pathological Fractures

1. False: it is caused not by a single traumatic incident but by repetitive minor stress.

2. False: it is a stress fracture of the metatarsals. A stress fracture of the fibula is known as 'runner's fracture'.

3. True: this may lead to spondylolisthesis.

4. False: they may be difficult to detect on X-rays, especially in the early stages. Later on a fracture line or periosteal new bone formation may be seen. Bone scan is the best method of early diagnosis.

5. False: they usually heal when the activity that caused them is stopped; however this may take many months.

6. True

7. True

8. True

9. False: often the underlying disorder needs medical treatment as well, e.g. osteomalacia, hyperparathyroidism, renal osteodystrophy and Paget's disease. Malignant conditions may need radiotherapy for palliation.

10. True

Injuries to Joints

1. Torn ligaments heal by fibrous scarring. (1)

2. Joints are usually unstable after ligaments sprains. (1)

3. Repair of a ruptured ligament is best delayed for 4 weeks until swelling has decreased. (1)

4. Subluxation implies complete dislocation of the articular surfaces of the joint. (1)

5. If the joint margins are damaged recurrent dislocation may follow. (1)

6. Following reduction of a dislocation, the joint should be moved as soon as possible. (1)

Total	6
Total score	
Postgraduate	6
Undergraduate	5

Answers opposite

Injuries to Joints

1. True

2. False

3. False: immediate repair gives better results.

4. False: subluxation is only partial dislocation.

5. True

6. False: it is best to rest the joint for 3–4 weeks to allow soft tissue damage to heal.

Injuries to the Upper Limb

1. Where does the clavicle usually fracture?(1)

2. What deformity of the clavicle arises and why?(1)

3. Fracture of the scapula normally requires internal fixation. (1)

4. In which direction does the shoulder normally dislocate?(1)

5. What two clinical findings should be noted before reducing a dislocated shoulder?(2)

6. Anterior dislocation of the shoulder often follows a blow from the posterior aspect. (1)

7. Acromioclavicular injury usually requires surgery. (1)

8. Anteroposterior radiographs of a posteriorly dislocated shoulder may be misleading. (1)

9. Epileptic fits or electric shock may give rise to posterior dislocation of the shoulder. (1)

10. Fractured neck of humerus commonly occurs in young people following a fall on to the outstretched hand. (1)

11. Accurate reduction of the fractured neck of humerus is essential in all cases. (1)

Answers opposite

Injuries of the Upper Limb

1. At the junction of the middle and outer thirds.

2. The distal fragment is pulled down by the weight of the arm and the proximal fragment is pulled upwards by the sternomastoid.

3. False: reduction is usually not required and the patient is allowed to mobilize as pain allows.

4. Anterior. This dislocation is approximately ten times more common than posterior dislocation.

5. The function of the axillary nerve and artery. These structures may be damaged during dislocation or reduction of the shoulder.

6. False: dislocation is commonly produced by a fall on the outstretched arm, driving the head of the humerus forward.

7. False: acromioclavicular joint injury is normally subluxation only and may be treated conservatively. Dislocation with wide displacement may require surgery.

8. True: if the dislocation is posterior, the humeral head remains at the same height and thus appears to be located in the glenoid on an isolated anteroposterior radiograph. A lateral radiograph should be taken to verify dislocation.

9. True: massive uncoordinated muscle spasm may cause posterior dislocation.

10. False: this fracture usually occurs in elderly osteoporotic women.

11. False: in elderly patients accurate reduction is not necessary and mobilization should commence as soon as pain allows.

12. Fractured shaft of humerus is nearly always spiral in nature due to the position of the nutrient artery entering the bone. (1)

13. The shaft of humerus is a recognized site for pathological fracture. (1)

14. What is the important neurological complication of fracture of the distal shaft of humerus?(1)

15. In supracondylar fracture of the humerus the distal fragment is displaced anteriorly. (1)

16. What is the most important immediate complication of supra-condylar fracture?(1)

17. Give two other complications of this injury. (2)

18. Before what age might fracture separation of the distal humeral epiphyses occur?(1)

19. Give four complications of elbow dislocation. (4)

20. The majority of fractured radial heads in adults are treated conservatively. (1)

21. Dislocation of the elbow is commonly anterior with the olecra-non slipping forward over the trochlea of the humerus. (1)

Answers opposite

12. False: commonly oblique and transverse fractures occur depending on the mode of injury. Spiral fractures follow a twisting force. The artery does not dictate the fracture pattern.

13. True: note the minimal force required to produce the fracture and the radiographic appearance which usually shows a lytic lesion.

14. Radial nerve palsy.

15. False: in 90% of cases the distal fragment displaces posteriorly.

16. Vascular damage to the brachial artery.

17. a) Compartment syndrome due to limb swelling and venous occlusion.
    b) Nerve injury – to the median nerve, rarely the ulnar or radial.
    c) Malunion – most commonly medial angulation to produce cubitus varus deformity.

18. Sixteen. After this age the humeral epiphyses fuse.

19. Vascular injury
    Nerve injury
    Stiffness (myositis ossificans)
    Tardy ulnar nerve palsy

20. True: treatment is usually 3 weeks in a sling with active flexion and extension being encouraged. Rarely, fractures with a single large fragment may be internally fixed.

21. False: it is most commonly posterior or posterolateral.

22. Myositis ossificans affects the whole limb after a viral illness. (1)

23. What are the two major symptoms of myositis ossificans?(2)

24. Open reduction and internal fixation is preferred in most displaced fractures of the forearm in adults. (1)

25. Compartment syndrome is not a complication of forearm fractures. (1)

26. Non-union of a single fractured forearm bone is a recognized complication. (1)

27. What is a Monteggia fracture?(1)

28. Colles's fracture is associated with osteoporosis. (1)

29. What is the position adopted by the distal radial fragment in Colles's fracture?(4)

30. Colles's fracture should be X-rayed at 1 week post fracture. (2)

Answers opposite

22. False: myositis ossificans is heterotopic ossification in the muscles and soft tissues around a joint following injury. It most commonly occurs at the elbow.

23. Increased pain after injury and limitation of movement in the recovery phase.

24. True: displacement occurs due to the rotational pull of the forearm muscles. Reduction and immobilization in plaster alone are often ineffective.

25. False: swelling of the soft tissues of the forearm within their deep fascia may give rise to compartment syndrome. Immediate decompression is warranted.

26. True: the intact forearm bone may splint the fractured bone apart, preventing union. Elective operative treatment may thus be preferred.

27. Monteggia fracture is a fracture of the upper ulna with the head of radius dislocated. The opposite fracture, Galeazzi, is fracture of the lower half of the radius with dislocation of the distal radioulnar joint.

28. True: it commonly occurs in elderly post-menopausal women after a fall on the outstretched hand.

29. Dorsal displacement
Dorsal angulation
Radial deviation
Impaction

30. True: redisplacement of the distal fragment may occur as the swelling of the wrist decreases and the plaster becomes loose.

31. Give three complications of Colles's fracture. (3)

32. A Smith's fracture is a 'reversed' Colles's fracture. (1)

33. Barton's fracture involves the ulna. (1)

34. Sudeck's atrophy describes weakness of the shoulder following injuries to the hand. (1)

35. Give one painful sign that helps with the clinical diagnosis of a fractured scaphoid. (1)

36. The middle portion of the scaphoid is most at risk of avascular necrosis following fracture because of its position. (1)

37. The anatomical snuff box is situated between the abductor pollicis longus and the flexor carpi radialis. (1)

38. Carpal dislocation often occurs around the lunate and is caused by forcible dorsiflexion. (1)

Answers opposite

31. Any three of:
Malunion
Tendon rupture
Stiffness
Sudeck's atrophy
Carpal tunnel syndrome
Subluxation of the radio-ulnar joint

32. True: the distal fragment is displaced in a volar direction.

33. False: Barton's fracture is a fracture of the distal radius which involves the articular surface of the wrist and the fracture fragment is displaced in a volar direction. It is a fracture-dislocation.

34. False: Sudeck's atrophy of the wrist and hand causes stiffness, pain and hypersensitivity. This troublesome condition may require prolonged treatment with physiotherapy and guanethidine nerve blocks.

35. One of the following:
Pain on dorsiflexion of the wrist
Tenderness in the anatomical snuff box
Pain on gripping with the affected hand

36. False: the proximal pole is most at risk because the nutrient artery to the scaphoid enters the bone distally and runs proximally. Fracture of the scaphoid may thus deprive the proximal pole of its blood supply.

37. False: it is between extensor pollicis longus and brevis.

38. True: the lunate is displaced anteriorly and must be reduced by open or closed reduction.

39. Bennett's fracture involves the proximal phalanx of the thumb. (1)

40. Which metacarpal is most often fractured and what is the usual mode of injury?(2)

41. Perilunate dislocation may be complicated by injury to which nerve?(1)

42. Rotational deformity may be safely ignored in metacarpal fractures. (1)

43. Gamekeeper's thumb is a chronic laxity of the ulnar collateral ligaments of the metacarpophalangeal joint of the thumb. (1)

44. If the hand has to be immobilized, what is the position of splintage?(1)

45. Because of the mobility of the hand, it rarely gets stiff when injured. (1)

46. Mallet finger follows the rupture of the extensor tendon to the distal phalanx. (1)

47. Isolated middle and ring finger metacarpal fractures rarely require internal fixation. (1)

48. A Smith's fracture takes 12 weeks to unite. (1)

Total score	61	
Target score		
Postgraduate	57	
Undergraduate	51	

Answers opposite

39. False: it is a fracture of the base of the 1st metacarpal. Treatment is by reduction and immobilization in plaster or internal fixation with a small screw.

40. The 5th metacarpal. Usually as a result of punching somebody or something.

41. Median nerve. This should be decompressed immediately.

42. False: failure to correct rotational deformity results in malalignment of the fingers in flexion.

43. True: due to wringing the necks of game birds.

44. Metacarpophalangeal joints at 90°. Interphalangeal joints at 0°.

45. False: the hand may get extremely stiff after injury, and to minimize this efforts should be made to reduce swelling, reduce the time in splintage and encourage early and active mobilization.

46. True

47. True: the fractured metacarpal is held out to length and held in position by the neighbouring unbroken metacarpals.

48. False: usually about 6 weeks.

Injuries of the Spine, Thorax, and Pelvis

1. In fractures of the spine classified as unstable, the spinal cord has been damaged. (1)

2. The primary factor in stability of the spine is the posterior ligament complex. (1)

3. Hangman's fracture is a fracture of the odontoid peg. (1)

4. Compression or crush fractures of the vertebral body are common in the elderly. (1)

5. Computerized tomography scanning is not as valuable as ultrasound in spinal fractures. (1)

6. Care of the bladder and skin to prevent urinary retention and pressure sores in the paraplegic patient should start 1 week following injury. (1)

7. Symptoms of 'whiplash' following a rear-end collision may persist for over a year. (1)

8. Wedge compression injury of the cervical spine follows extension and rotation forces. (1)

9. Dislocation of the cervical facet joints cannot occur without a fracture. (1)

10. Unilateral facet dislocation of the cervical spine is rarely associated with spinal cord injury. (1)

11. Crush fractures of the cervical spine are rarely complicated by cord damage. (1)

12. Following compression fracture of the thoracolumbar spine, patients may require 3 months in plaster. (1)

Answers opposite

Injuries of the Spine, Thorax, and Pelvis

1. False: the unstable classification refers to the nature of the fracture which may displace and subsequently damage the spinal cord.

2. True

3. False: it is a fracture of the pedicles of C2 vertebra.

4. True: due to osteoporosis.

5. False: computerized tomography scanning is of great value in showing fractures of the neural arch or encroachment of the spinal cord. Ultrasound is extremely limited.

6. False: pressure sores may develop within 2 hours of injury if the patient is left in the same position.

7. True: although the pathology is unclear.

8. False: it is caused by hyperflexion.

9. False: unilateral or bilateral facet joint dislocation may occur without a fracture.

10. True: unilateral facet dislocation rarely allows forward subluxation of more than one third of the vertebral body, thus the cord is rarely compressed.

11. False: fragments are often driven back into the spinal canal producing cord damage.

12. True

13. The thoracolumbar junction is the most common site for flexion rotation injuries. (1)

14. Spinal shock may last for 3 months. (1)

15. Cauda equina injury results in spastic paralysis and exaggerated reflexes below the level of the lesion. (1)

16. The anal reflex is lost in complete cord transection at the level of T10. (1)

17. Pressure sores rarely develop in areas of anaesthetic skin. (1)

18. Paralysed limbs become hypermobile and floppy after 3 months. (1)

19. Heterotopic ossification occurs in paralysed limbs. (1)

20. General anaesthesia by intubation and ventilation is contraindicated in patients who have multiple rib fractures and a flail segment.

21. A patient with a tension pneumothorax due to a fractured rib should be re-X-rayed at 24-hour intervals to observe resolution. (1)

22. Fractures of the pelvic ring are rarely complicated by genitourinary damage. (1)

23. Segments of bone avulsed from the pelvis by violent muscle contraction should be replaced and internally fixed. (1)

24. Fractures of the pubic rami are common following falls in elderly persons. (1)

Answers opposite

13. True

14. False: if the complete paralysis of spinal shock persists for more than 48 hours recovery does not occur and the neural deficit becomes permanent.

15. False: the cauda equina lesion is a lower motor neurone injury and results in flaccid paralysis.

16. False

17. False: anaesthetic skin is extremely vulnerable.

18. False: without regular passive movement, they develop flexion contractures.

19. True: the mechanism is unclear.

20. False: positive pressure ventilation is in fact an effective method of treatment.

21. False: tension pneumothorax is a surgical emergency and should be decompressed immediately.

22. False: approximately 20% suffer genitourinary injury.

23. False: these are essentially muscular injuries only and should be treated by rest.

24. True: they are due to osteoporosis, and require symptomatic treatment only.

25. A break in the pelvic ring indicates pelvic instability. (1)

26. Fractures of the pelvic ring may be associated with massive blood loss and severe shock. (1)

27. Visceral damage to spleen and liver may occur by the same injury which produces pelvic fracture. (1)

28. Peritoneal lavage indicates the possibility of retroperitoneal bleeding following pelvic ring fracture. (1)

29. Repair to urogenital damage complicating pelvic fractures should be carried out as an emergency. (1)

30. Anterior fracture of the acetabulum is associated with a good prognosis. (1)

31. Open reduction of fractures of the posterior acetabulum should be undertaken if closed reduction is unsuccessful. (1)

32. What investigation is useful in complex fractures of the acetabulum in addition to plain radiographs? (1)

33. Avascular necrosis may follow posterior dislocation of the femoral head. (1)

34. Injuries to the coccyx resolve rapidly within days. (1)

Total	34
Target score	
Postgraduate	30
Undergraduate	26

Answers opposite

25. False: the pelvis is usually stable unless the sacroiliac elements are disrupted.

26. True: immediate resuscitation should commence.

27. True

28. False: peritoneal lavage will diagnose only intra-abdominal bleeding.

29. False: urinary drainage should be established and expert urethral repair carried out as an elective procedure.

30. True: anterior fractures do not affect the weight bearing area of the acetabulum.

31. True: inadequate reduction will lead to post-traumatic osteoarthritis.

32. Computerized tomography scanning.

33. True: due to disruption of the capsular blood supply.

34. False

Injuries to the Lower Limb

1. Traumatic dislocations of the hip are usually anterior. (1)

2. Hip dislocation is commonly associated with fracture of the femur. (1)

3. Computerized tomography scans are usually unhelpful in the diagnosis of acetabular fractures associated with traumatic dislocation of the hip. (1)

4. Hip dislocation requires open reduction. (1)

5. The sciatic nerve is usually injured in posterior hip dislocation. (1)

6. The blood supply to the femoral head is seriously impaired in 20% of traumatic hip dislocations. (1)

7. Anterior dislocation of the hip is easily diagnosed clinically. (1)

8. Secondary osteoarthritis is common after central dislocation of the hip. (1)

9. The Brooke–Taylor system is commonly used to classify femoral neck fractures. (1)

10. Femoral neck fractures in elderly women may both cause and be caused by a fall. (1).

11. Impacted fractures of the femoral neck are more painful than displaced fractures. (1)

12. The characteristic position of the leg following femoral neck fractures is short and internally rotated. (1)

Answers opposite

Injuries of the Lower Limb

1. False: four out of five are posterior.

2. False: but when they do occur together the hip dislocation is often missed on clinical examination. X-rays of all cases of femoral fractures should therefore include the pelvis.

3. False: they are almost essential as they often show up fragments that cannot be seen on plain X-rays.

4. False: most may be reduced closed under general anaesthetic. Associated femoral fractures and acetabular fractures may require open reduction and internal fixation.

5. False: fortunately this complication is not common but it must be carefully looked for in each case.

6. True: avascular necrosis and collapse is therefore a serious potential complication.

7. True: the dislocated femoral head is clearly seen as an anterior bulge.

8. True

9. False: the standard classification is that of Garden.

10. True

11. False: the opposite is generally true and some patients even walk around on impacted fractures.

12. False: it is short and externally or laterally rotated.

13. Displaced fractures of the femoral neck have a high incidence of non-union and avascular necrosis. (1)

14. Undisplaced femoral neck fractures should be treated with prosthetic femoral head replacement. (1)

15. Displaced femoral neck fractures in young people should be reduced and internally fixed. (1)

16. Early mobilization should be encouraged in the elderly following surgery to femoral neck fractures. (1)

17. Secondary osteoarthritis may occur immediately following avascular necrosis of the femoral head. (1)

18. Intertrochanteric fractures are common in young adults. (1)

19. The characteristic position of the leg following intertrochanteric fracture is short and externally rotated. (1)

20. Intertrochanteric fractures commonly fail to unite if they are not internally fixed. (1)

21. Avascular necrosis and femoral head collapse is a recognized complication of intertrochanteric fracture. (1)

22. Malunited intertrochanteric fractures seldom require further treatment. (1)

23. Spiral fractures of the femur are usually caused by direct blows. (1)

24. Pathological fractures of the femoral shaft are more likely in the elderly. (1)

Answers opposite

13. True

14. False: undisplaced fractures (Garden 1 or 2) have a relatively good prognosis and can be treated by internal fixation.

15. True: in the over 60s these fractures are usually treated by excision of the femoral head and insertion of a prosthesis, e.g. Thompson's or Austin Moore's hemiarthroplasty.

16. True: prolonged bed rest results in complications.

17. False: if secondary osteoarthritis occurs it is usually several years following avascular necrosis.

18. False: like femoral neck fractures they are commonest in elderly osteoporotic women.

19. True

20. False: they unite readily but are usually internally fixed with a sliding screw and plate in order to obtain the best possible position and to get the patient walking as soon as possible.

21. False

22. True

23. False: they are usually caused by twisting injuries.

24. True

25. Shock and fat embolism are common complications of femoral shaft fractures. (1)

26. The pelvis should always be X-rayed in cases of femoral shaft fractures. (1)

27. Closed treatment of femoral fractures is more satisfactory in fractures of the proximal third than the distal third. (1)

28. Femoral fractures in children can usually be treated with skin traction. (1)

29. The most satisfactory method of internal fixation of femoral shaft fractures in adults is with a long plate. (1)

30. Intramedullary fixation of femoral fractures allows early movement of hip and knee. (1)

31. Up to half a litre of blood can be lost with a closed femoral shaft fracture. (1)

32. A fractured femur should unite in 100 days, plus or minus 20. (1)

33. Malunion of up to 15° of femoral shaft fractures may go unnoticed. (1)

34. The knee is seldom affected in femoral shaft fractures. (1)

35. In supracondylar fractures of the femur the distal fragment tends to rotate forwards. (1)

36. Conservative treatment of supracondylar femoral fractures can be effectively achieved from the outset with a cast brace. (1)

Answers opposite

25. True

26. True

27. False: control of the small proximal fragment in proximal third fractures is often difficult.

28. True

29. False: intramedullary nails give better biomechanical stability. To improve rotational stability and to prevent shortening occurring in comminuted fractures, interlocking screws can be added proximally and distally.

30. True

31. False: the figure is closer to 1½ litres.

32. True

33. True

34. False: it may be injured at the same time as the femoral fracture or it may stiffen because of soft tissue adhesions during treatment.

35. False: in this injury the gastrocnemius rotates the distal fragment posteriorly.

36. False: the cast brace is only of use when the fracture is beginning to unite at approximately 4–6 weeks. Prior to this traction or splintage is necessary.

37. Internal fixation of supracondylar fractures is often difficult because of osteoporosis. (1)

38. Haemarthrosis is a rare but serious complication of femoral condylar fractures. (1)

39. Knee stiffness is common following condylar fractures. (1)

40. Depressed tibial plateau fractures usually require surgical elevation and internal fixation. (1)

41. The lateral tibial plateau is more commonly fractured than the medial. (1)

42. Stellate patella fractures are usually associated with a rupture of the extensor mechanism. (1)

43. A congenital bipartite patella can easily be confused with a transverse fracture of the patella. (1)

44. Surgical repair is essential in displaced transverse patellar fractures. (1)

45. Patella dislocation is usually to the medial side of the knee. (1)

46. Genu valgum predisposes to patella dislocation. (1)

47. Collateral ligament injuries of the knee are more common on the medial side. (1)

48. Complete collateral ligament tears of the knee are more painful than partial tears. (1)

49. Swelling of the knee is worse with partial than complete ligament tears. (1)

Answers opposite

37. True

38. False: it is almost always present and is not in itself very serious.

39. True

40. True

41. True

42. False: the extensor mechanism is usually intact with stellate fractures but disrupted with displaced transverse fractures.

43. False: in a congenital bipartite patella the line between the two fragments is usually obliquely across the superolateral angle of the bone, not transverse.

44. True: to reconstitute the extensor mechanism.

45. False: it is lateral in almost every case.

46. True

47. True

48. False

49. True: this is because in complete tears the capsule is disrupted and any joint effusion can escape.

50. The Lachman test shows up a ruptured medial collateral ligament. (1)

51. Anterior cruciate laxity may be treated by reattachment, reinforcement or replacement. (1)

52. Knee dislocation can occur after minor injury. (1)

53. Motor cycle accidents are the most common cause of tibia and fibula fractures. (1)

54. Closed fractures of the tibia and fibula can be satisfactorily treated by plaster. (1)

55. Isolated fractures of the tibia are prone to non-union. (1)

56. Stress fracture of the tibia is common in army recruits. (1)

57. Ankle sprains can be treated by active mobilization in a crêpe bandage. (1)

58. Complete tears of ankle ligaments must be surgically repaired. (1)

59. In recurrent lateral ligament instability of the ankle, reconstruction may be undertaken using the peroneus longus tendon. (1)

60. External rotation injuries of the ankle result in an oblique fracture of the lateral malleolus and a transverse fracture of the medial malleolus. (1)

61. Adduction injuries of the ankle result in an oblique fracture of the medial malleolus and a ruptured lateral ligament or transverse fracture of the lateral malleolus. (1)

Answers opposite

50. False: it tests the cruciate ligaments, particularly the anterior cruciate.

51. True

52. False: this is a rare injury requiring a force of considerable magnitude.

53. True

54. True

55. True: the intact fibula may hold the ends apart. If this occurs then the fibula may need to be divided.

56. True: due to prolonged marching.

57. True

58. False: plaster immobilization is satisfactory in most cases.

59. False: peroneus brevis is usually used.

60. True

61. True

62. Ankle fractures can result in fibular fractures anywhere between ankle and knee. (1)

63. Fractures of both medial and lateral malleoli where the fibula fracture is above the inferior tibiofibular joint can be satisfactorily treated in plaster. (1)

64. Ankles should always be immobilized in equinus. (1)

65. Talar fractures may be complicated by avascular necrosis of the head. (1)

66. Calcaneal fractures are usually sustained by forced dorsiflexion of the ankle. (1)

67. Calcaneal fractures seldom cause osteoarthritis of the ankle joint. (1)

68. The calcaneus can be clearly seen in anteroposterior and lateral ankle X-rays. (1)

69. Metatarsal fractures usually heal readily but require a plaster for comfort. (1)

70. Fractures of the toes are best treated with a weight bearing plaster of Paris cast. (1)

Total score	70
Target score	
Postgraduate	64
Undergraduate	55

Answers opposite

True

 3. False: this injury is unstable and usually requires open reduction and internal fixation.

64. False: this should be avoided or contractures of the joint and the Achilles tendon may occur.

65. False: it is the body that is prone to undergo avascular necrosis not the head.

66. False: they are usually sustained by falls from a height, often from a ladder. They are associated with fractures of the hip, pelvis, and spine.

67. True: they do, however, cause osteoarthritis of the subtalar joints and if disability is severe, fusion of the subtalar joint may be needed.

68. False: special calcaneal views should be taken.

69. True

70. False: isolated fractures of the toes are best left unsplinted and the patient encouraged to walk.